ACDF
ANTERIOR CERVICAL DISCECTOMY AND FUSION

The Informed Patient

ACDF
ANTERIOR CERVICAL DISCECTOMY AND FUSION

The Informed Patient

My Journey Undergoing Neck Fusion Surgery

Patrick O. Smith

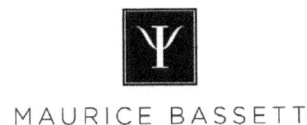

MAURICE BASSETT

ACDF: The Informed Patient. My journey undergoing neck fusion surgery

Copyright © 2020 by Maurice Bassett

All rights reserved. No part of this book may be reproduced or copied in any form without written permission from the publisher.

Maurice Bassett
P.O. Box 839
Anna Maria, FL 34216

Contact the publisher:
MauriceBassett@gmail.com
www.MauriceBassett.com

Contact the author:
www.NeckFusionSurgery.com

Cover design and interior illustration: David Michael Moore
Editing and interior layout: Chris Nelson

ISBN: 978-1-60025-163-4

Library of Congress Control Number: 2020947514

Important note: The information, opinions and suggestions in this book DO NOT CONSTITUTE MEDICAL ADVICE. The author is sharing his personal experience and research in the hopes that readers will become more informed on their own personal journey. The author is not a medical professional. Nothing in this book should be taken as professional advice, and neither the publisher nor the author will be liable for any consequences or damages arising directly or indirectly from the use of this book.

In consideration of full disclosure, none of the physicians, products, or companies mentioned in this book have received any type of endorsements, compensation or other incentives whatsoever.

Original names and identifying details of many of the individuals appearing in this book have been changed to protect the privacy of individuals.

Dedications

This book is dedicated to my wife Jennifer and to Mateusz Zagata, M.D., who did not give up on me during my times of sickness or health.

My wife has shown her love for me through her relentless acts of service and patience, and she continues to do so.

Dr. Zagata is the epitome of what a physician should be. He does what he is called to do and embodies the oath he took to care for those who suffer. Dr. Zagata is truly a servant of God of the highest calling. It is by no coincidence that I have come to know him.

Contents

Foreword by Mateusz Zagata, M.D. 11

Chapter 1: What is ACDF? 15
    Becoming an Informed Patient 18
    Be Your Own Advocate 20

Chapter 2: Case History 23
    The Accident 23
    Understanding Your Own Injuries 26
    Signs and Symptoms 27

Chapter 3: Initial Diagnosis 29
    Easing the Pain Between Appointments 30
    Specialist Referral 30
    Problems with Diagnostic Testing 38
    The Role of the Radiologist 39

Chapter 4: Surgical Consultation 41
    The Choice of a Surgeon 41
    My First Surgical Consultation 42
    Seeking a Second Opinion 42
    Neurosurgeon or Orthopedic Surgeon? 43
    The Second Surgical Consultation 45
    Questioning the Doctor 46
    The Implant 46

Allograft 48
Before Surgery and Pre-Operative Consultation 50
Blood Testing 50
Anesthesiologist 51

Chapter 5: Surgery and Post-Op 53
Post-operative Recovery 54
Dysphasia 55
Pain 56
The Day After 57
Neck Brace 59
Going Home 59
Recovery 60

Chapter 6: Understanding and Managing Pain 63
The Nature of Pain 63
Pain and the Informed Patient 64
Post-op ACDF Adjustment-Phase Pain 65
Pain Scales 66
Physician Choice: General Practitioner or Specialist? 66
Coping and Family Support 68

Chapter 7: Pain Management Modalities 71
Many Modalities: What Works for You? 71
Medications 72
Prescription and OTC Pain Medications 72
Opioids 74
Medical Marijuana and Other Medications 76
Non-Medication Treatments 77

Myofascial Release Therapy 77
Nerve Ablation and Nerve Blocks 78
Physical Therapy and the McKenzie Method of Mechanical Diagnosis and Therapy 79
Cognitive Behavioral Therapy 82
Lifestyle, Exercise and Diet 83
Cold/hot Showers 84
Acupressure Mat 84
TENS Units 85
Cold Laser Therapy 85
Conclusion 85

Chapter 8: Health Insurance **87**
Health Insurance Companies 87
Read Your Policy 88
Pre-authorization 89
Advocate for Yourself 90

Chapter 9: Medical Privacy **93**

Chapter 10: Healthy Living **97**

Chapter 11: Reflections on Being an Informed Patient **101**

Glossary **103**

Index **111**

Acknowledgments **125**

About the Author **127**

Foreword

Mateusz Zagata, M.D.

As a board certified physician specializing in family medicine it is my job to treat and ease the suffering of all the patients I see to the best of my ability, for any condition. I am usually the first line of contact and help for many patients seeking treatment. This includes neck and back pain and injury, one of America's most common debilitating conditions. Once a preliminary diagnosis has been made, I may refer the patient to a specialist for further treatment, which may include surgery. Many of the patients needing surgery for spinal conditions usually end up coming back to see me for pain management and related issues post-operative. Unfortunately, for reasons out of our control, we do not always have the time we want to spend with patients who seek out detailed information about their condition, and some patients simply don't want to know. As a physician I am responsible for a patient's care and well-being throughout the treatment process, which may include post-operative care. Part of my consultation involves answering patient questions, and I spend a lot of time doing just that. Although physicians do their best to keep patients informed and comfortable throughout the process, we are each, of course, only one person—and we have many patients. Furthermore, patients who undergo any type of surgery are subject to new experiences, and often new questions arise.

In this book, Patrick does a wonderful job explaining his

experiences undergoing cervical spinal fusion surgery from a patient's perspective. Fortunately, I have never had to undergo spinal fusion surgery. I think this book will not only help patients understand the process of undergoing anterior cervical discectomy and fusion surgery (ACDF), but may also be useful to anyone in the medical field who treats such patients.

As Patrick descriptively points out, it is important to become an informed patient for your own sake and for the sake of your family. So take the time to become an informed patient. Ask the right questions and educate yourself on the process of undergoing anterior cervical discectomy and fusion surgery if the procedure is recommended by your surgeon. I agree with Patrick that being an "informed patient" will benefit you, your family and your health.

Mateusz Zagata, M.D.

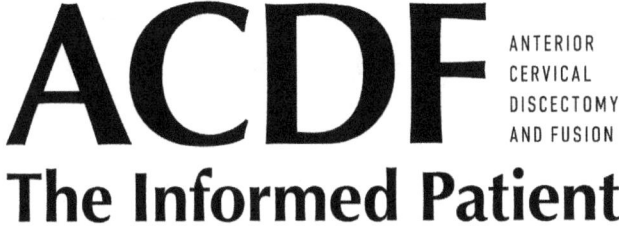

> "Everyone has a doctor in him or her;
> We just have to help it in its work.
> The natural healing force within each of us
> Is the greatest force in getting well."
> ~ Hippocrates

Chapter 1

What is ACDF?

July, 2006.

I vaguely remember voices in the background trying to determine how to get me to the hospital. An emergency medical helicopter? An ambulance?

I'd crashed my dirt-bike motorcycle on a local racing track. My friends and the track staff found me unconscious, and later recognized that I was in shock. They knew I needed medical attention right away. In the end they transported me to the hospital via ambulance.

It was later determined that I'd sustained a fractured pelvis in four separate locations, several fractured ribs, a fractured collar bone and a severe concussion—not to mention bruises along the entire length of my body. What wasn't discovered during my initial assessment by the attending physician were three ruptured cervical discs.

Over the course of the next six years I would slowly and painfully learn that I needed to undergo ACDF (anterior cervical discectomy and fusion) surgery, commonly known as neck fusion surgery.

That's where this story really begins.

***

In the Spring of 2012, six years after my accident on the dirt-bike track, I sought further treatment. I'd been experiencing low, dull, chronic neck pain, as well as radiating arm pain, numbness and tingling in my right hand. I wanted a proper diagnosis to see what I could do about it. After referral to and surgical consultation with my orthopedic spine surgeon in 2013, I was recommended for anterior cervical discectomy and fusion with instrumentation surgery, also known as ACDF. In layman's terms it's called "neck fusion surgery."

ACDF surgery was developed in the 1950s out of a need to treat Pott's disease,[1] a form of tuberculosis that affects the vertebrae. Since then, ACDF has become the gold standard for cervical surgery for trauma-related injuries and degenerative disc pathology, as well as for other conditions. ACDF is one of the most common spinal surgeries performed today; over one million ACDF surgeries were performed in the U.S. between 2006 and 2013.[2] ACDF surgery involves removing a damaged disc from the spinal column and replacing it with a "spacer" bone graft or the use of a prosthetic device that helps fuse together the vertebrae above and below the removed disc. We will explore this process in greater detail later in the book.

As a patient beginning this journey, I wanted to become informed about the process. I began researching information on what to expect during my upcoming surgery and post-operative recovery. I quickly realized that there was limited information available for patients undergoing ACDF surgery, both on the process itself as well as from diagnostic and post-operative recovery perspectives. In general, the

---

[1] Leven, Dante, and Samuel K. Cho. "Pseudarthrosis of the Cervical Spine: Risk Factors, Diagnosis and Management." Asian Spine Journal, Korean Society of Spine Surgery, Aug. 2016, www.ncbi.nlm.nih.gov/pmc/articles/PMC4995265/
[2] Saifi C, Fein AW, Cazzulino A, et al. Trends in resource utilization and rate of cervical disc arthroplasty and anterior cervical discectomy and fusion throughout the United States from 2006 to 2013. *Spine J.* 2018;18(6):1022-1029. doi:10.1016/j.spinee.2017.10.072

material I found on ACDF surgery was either technical surgical literature written for medical students and physicians or, if drawn from various internet sources, was limited, subjective, and at times inaccurate.

Internet searches led me to spinal fusion chat rooms, community boards, and medical industry-fueled advertisements. Although some of the information was truly informative, it did not tell the entire story, which is what I wanted to know: what to expect from diagnosis through post-operative recovery. What I did learn is that, as mentioned above, ACDF surgery is a very common medical procedure. I also learned that many people suffer from post-operative pain and psychological setbacks after undergoing ACDF surgery.

Throughout this book I share my own insights and experiences, as well as offering explanations for medical terms associated with ACDF surgery, treatment, and post-op recovery. At the end of the book I also include a glossary of medical terminology most commonly associated with ACDF surgery and treatment to assist with deciphering the technical language used by the medical community.

My prior work experience, training, and education as an Emergency Medical Technician (EMT) tending to trauma victims has helped me decipher and understand the medical processes and jargon that a patient will encounter while exploring ACDF surgery. Nonetheless, only an experienced medical doctor (M.D.), physician's assistant (P.A.), advanced practice registered nurse (A.P.R.N.) or other person possessing the equivalent specialized medical training is qualified to make a proper diagnosis and give medical advice or treatment. This book is based on my personal experiences and research as an informed patient who has undergone ACDF surgery, and is no substitute for professional medical advice or diagnosis.

With that said, I do hope that it will help as a guide along the way while you seek out the professional support you need.

Becoming an Informed Patient

I also hope this book helps current and prospective ACDF patients become informed patients so that they can live happier and healthier lives. You owe it to yourself and your family to seek out the right information and learn to ask the right questions prior to ACDF surgery so that you can learn how to live comfortably after it. The dangers of being an uninformed patient are too great a risk.

As I did research for this book, both prior to my own surgery and afterwards, I was amazed to discover how little many ACDF patients and prospective patients know about their own condition, sometimes even after they've had the surgery. (As a side note, most members of the "ACDF club" become experts at recognizing other members. From the tell-tale surgical scars on the throat to the constant stretching and massaging of the neck, it becomes clear as to who has undergone ACDF surgery.)

Before and after my own surgery I spoke to several people who had either undergone or were considering undergoing ACDF surgery. I hoped to gain some sort of information and insight into the process. I also wanted to learn how they managed their pre and post-operative pain and discomfort. I found that many did not have enough information to properly cope with their pain and discomfort. Several of the people I spoke with were ill-informed, confused, or just not interested in knowing about their own condition or about ACDF surgery. Many were suffering from severe to moderate pain and taking potent prescription pain medication to cope. I think this is a dangerous position to be in as an ACDF patient. I understand that perhaps some patients simply don't want to know what they are facing, or are too scared to think about all the things that can go wrong—or are even in complete denial. But my own feeling is that it's usually better to be informed in detail about what to expect from beginning to end. Patients should not go through this procedure blindly.

Individuals who don't inform themselves about the basic concepts of ACDF surgery and what to expect during recovery are limiting their control over the procedure itself and their quality of care. And being an uninformed patient can affect long-term care options and quality of life, not to mention the cost associated with care. In my experience, an uninformed patient increases his or her chances of becoming frustrated with the post-operative conditions resulting from ACDF surgery, including having a lack of insight into how to eliminate or reduce pre-operative and post-operative pain and suffering. Patients should at least be aware of the many different types of treatment modalities which might best suit them to assist with their recovery.

Many patients do not fully comprehend the significance of their condition or the seriousness of ACDF surgery. Although the procedure may seem straightforward and normal to an orthopedic spine surgeon who conducts hundreds of ACDF surgeries a year, patients need to know it is an invasive surgery with many associated potential risks, including death, paralysis, hemorrhage, carotid artery damage, nerve damage, infection, failure of fusion (pseudarthrosis), mechanical failure and a host of other possible complications.

Patients should be made fully aware of all associated risks. This responsibility should perhaps rest on the medical professionals and the insurance companies who provide related medical care and advisement. But ultimately it's the patients (and their families) who must live with resulting conditions following ACDF surgery. So it only makes sense that patients should be well-informed and know as much as possible ahead of time about ACDF surgery.

Be Your Own Advocate

Why is it important to be your own advocate? The risks to your health during any major medical procedure are too great not to be. Within the medical community things go wrong all the time. Although most mistakes and unexpected occurrences are not life-threatening and are easily corrected, they sometimes become part of a chain of events that can lead to a patient's death or debilitating injury. Sometimes details are overlooked even during medical and surgical procedures.

Why? The answer is simple: because there are hundreds of decisions being made throughout the process leading up to and including surgery and recovery. A *lot* of people are involved in making those decisions, from healthcare professionals to patients to hospital administrators to insurance companies. From the time you walk into your GP's office through post-operative recovery, hundreds of people are involved directly or indirectly in your care. And everyone plays an important role in their own way, whether they're an administrative clerk, nurses' aide, registered nurse, physician's assistant, technician, radiologist, anesthesiologist, respiratory therapist, physical therapist, medical doctor or other specialist. Even the hospital custodians wage germ warfare on a daily basis to protect patients from infectious diseases.

Of course, most people tend to get comfortable in their roles, and this sometimes leads to complacency. This complacency can result in accidentally overlooking important details. Did the nurse or doctor note down all relevant patient details in the chart? Did the insurance company approve the procedure correctly? Did the radiologist read the MRI accurately? These and other issues can have dire consequences for a patient's physical and financial health if they are not handled correctly.

That's why being an informed patient is the best way to prepare for ACDF surgery—or for any other major healthcare procedure, for that matter. Especially if you are going to be incoherent or unconscious at some point (as you will be when undergoing ACDF surgery), it should be made mandatory to have a patient liaison to accompany you throughout the process. A patient liaison can be a family member or someone appointed by the hospital or medical facility to assist you while you are unconscious or under the influence of medication before, during and after medical procedures. They can act as your advocate with respect to your personal health decisions.

Being a good advocate for yourself also includes maintaining documentation. This can be exceptionally helpful especially when things go wrong. It's always important to retain copies of every piece of communication while collecting specific hospital records, and also during the administration and processing of paperwork for the insurance company. This includes any and all forms of documentation that you sign—and *do* make sure to request copies. Keep detailed records and notes of phone conversations, including the names of the people with whom you speak, and the dates and times. This can be important not only should something go wrong, but also when making insurance claims.

In short, it's always better to be an informed patient. Even if you don't know the inner workings of the medical community or have difficulty interpreting medical language, you can at least do your best to educate yourself on the basics. I hope this book serves as a step in that direction. At a minimum, asking the right questions will help you further understand what to expect when undergoing ACDF surgery. And if you don't have as much time as you need to investigate, at least ask a friend or family member to assist you along the way. Your health depends on it.

Chapter 2

Case History

The Accident

During the summer of 2006 I was involved in a motocross accident that left me unconscious and with a fractured pelvis. It also led me straight to the emergency room. The accident involved a traumatic, high-speed impact fall from a great height. I landed on my side on a compact clay and dirt surface. I cannot say for certain if this single incident was the cause of my subsequent ongoing cervical neck pain and related ACDF surgery, but I'm sure it greatly contributed. Luckily, at the time of my accident I was wearing a helmet and protective gear. Had this not been the case, things could have been much worse.

    I was unconscious and in shock for several minutes following the accident. My friend and the track staff drove me dazed and confused via golf cart back to our tent staging area. (This was probably not the best course of action for a motor vehicle accident victim with suspected cervical trauma. Haphazardly moving a patient with cervical injuries can inflict further damage and cause severe injury, paralysis, or death.)

    I was later transported via ambulance to a local hospital after my friend recognized that I was experiencing symptoms of shock and confusion. I do not remember the ambulance ride or being brought into the ER. I can only recall some of the events that happened prior to and after the accident. Most of what I learned about my accident came from the friends, family and first responders who had witnessed it.

During my visit to the ER, the attending physician interviewed a friend of mine who had seen the accident. This is a good point to remember: having a witness help medical personnel determine exactly what happened during an accident can be extremely helpful for guiding patient treatment and care. The doctor also conducted an initial assessment and manual exam, as well as taking X-rays and MRIs (Magnetic Resonance Imaging) of my lower spine, pelvic region, and head.

At that time, the MRI images taken of my head were limited to the C3 (cervical vertebrae 3) level—just above the injured area. So unfortunately these images did not reveal any potentially injured discs or cervical bones below the C3 level.

The cervical spine is made up of seven vertebrae, with vertebral discs in between each vertebra (see illustration on page 25). The injuries sustained to my neck between C3-C4, C5-C6, and C6-C7 went undiagnosed mainly for two reasons: 1) I did not complain of neck pain and 2) the MRI taken of my head did not show the lower cervical vertebrae.[3]

After the shock wore off and the pain from my injuries began to set in, I was administered the pain medication Demerol for the onset of acute pain. My family members were instructed to monitor me for post-concussion MTBI (mild traumatic brain injury) and internal bleeding symptoms.

---

[3] As a side note, an emergency room is very often an extremely fast-paced environment in which an attending physician must jump from patient to patient to quickly assess the severity of injuries and—simply put—try to make sure no one dies. In this setting, things can get "missed," but I consider missing a few bulging discs a minor event when I consider that my pelvis was broken in four places and I had a fracture along a femoral artery that was potentially life-threatening.

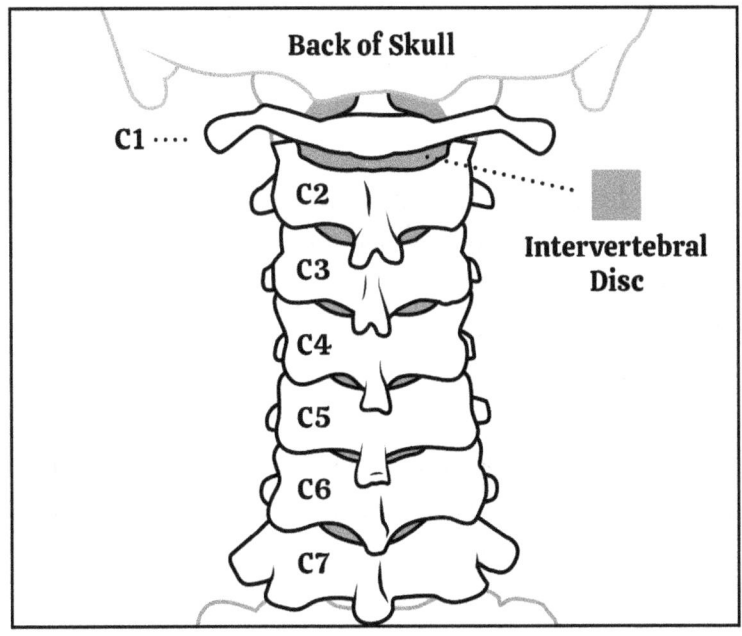

After receiving medical care at the ER, I was released with the determination that there was no need for surgical intervention. Because I was experiencing symptoms of a concussion and in shock when brought in to the ER, I did not participate in the patient history and assessment portion of my ER visit. Follow-up appointments with an orthopedic physician and my primary care physician (PCP) were made after the accident to ensure my pelvis was healing properly and that post-concussion safety measures were being taken. I was prescribed Vicodin brand pain medication, also known as dihydrocodeine (a semi-synthetic opioid synthesized from codeine and one of the opioid alkaloids found in the opium poppy) for my post-accident pain. Hydrocodone (generic Vicodin) is used to treat acute and severe chronic pain. This was only my second time ever having been prescribed an opioid-based pain medication, and it was my first time being prescribed one for an extended length of time during my recovery phase. Later I will discuss the benefits and dangers of opioid-based analgesic pain medication.

Understanding Your Own Injuries

Although I did not complain of neck pain immediately after my accident, I suspect most of my neck injuries were sustained at that time. Over the next six years the insidiously slow onset and presentation of referred pain in my neck and shoulders left me without immediate answers as to why my neck was in constant pain. I did not consider, nor realize until years later, that much of the pain I was experiencing may have been due to my accident. On the other hand, throughout my younger years I was involved in all sorts of accidents and sustained numerous injuries, including bicycle and skiing accidents, falls from skateboards and a fall from a tree. It's quite possible that any of these accidents also caused some sort of trauma to my neck.

Obviously, it can help in the diagnosis and treatment phases to understand, if possible, *why* your neck hurts. Many injuries to the cervical vertebrae and discs are misdiagnosed as muscle sprains and tears. If you do have some idea about why and when your pain started, make sure to share this information with your physician. It can be helpful to think about this prior to your first appointment rather than trying to remember "on the spot" in the short time you have with your doctor. Even if you can't pinpoint with certainty when something happened, you might come up with some pieces of the puzzle for a doctor to consider. My own history of accidents indicated that there were several potential causes for my pain, with the likeliest culprit being my dirt bike accident. So if you have the details of an accident or injury at hand to share with your physician, this can be helpful information in the diagnostic and treatment process.

It's also true that newer imaging technology and detailed patient assessments allow physicians to make better-informed decisions as to the cause of pain and injury in a given case. Having an experienced physician is just as important as the technology. Without an experienced physician, injuries may go undiagnosed and cause further complications, not the least of which is ongoing discomfort and pain for the patient. Luckily, when I eventually put two and two together and decided to talk with my family physician in 2013, he quickly and accurately assessed what I was experiencing and immediately put me on a course of treatment. I will explain more about this in the next chapter.

Signs and Symptoms

Fast forward six years after the accident. My first neck pain symptoms appeared in the summer of 2012, though they may have manifested intermittently over the preceding years as a deep muscle ache, a more subtle neck pain. In early 2013 I became more aware of a pain that presented on the right side of my neck and radiated into my right shoulder, extending into my arm and hand. I've always carried tension and stress in my neck and shoulder area, so the constant, annoying pain was familiar. One of the problems resulting from the slow onset of my many symptoms from disc degeneration, disc protrusion, nerve impingement, arthritis and stenosis is that I did not recognize what was happening, and this slowed my diagnosis and treatment.

Usually, upon feeling the onset of this dull, annoying ache I would manually massage my neck or ask a family member to do so for me, as well as take over-the-counter (OTC) pain-relieving medication. The medications I found to be most beneficial in relieving this type of low-level pain were acetaminophen, better known as Tylenol, and ibuprofen, brand name Advil (an NSAID, or nonsteroidal anti-inflammatory drug). These medications and massages helped to ease the annoying dull ache that never seemed to go away entirely.

As time went on the pain became increasingly more intense and unbearable. A few days prior to my diagnosis I had a painful neck and shoulder episode for which I sought relief from a local massage therapist. I was hoping that a professional, licensed massage therapist could provide immediate help and give my family a break from my constant complaining. During my initial consultation with the massage therapist I made it very clear that I wanted them to focus on my neck and shoulder area and to apply a lot of pressure. In the past I'd found it extremely frustrating when I wanted to get a massage to relieve pain and the therapist didn't apply enough pressure to break up what I thought was myofascial pain or a muscle spasm.

But after getting my neck and shoulders massaged by the therapist I realized that I was in more pain than when I had gone in. Because I demanded a lot of pressure be applied, the massage more than likely caused the cervical nerves to become irritated and inflamed. The force applied to loosen the muscles in my neck likely exacerbated already irritated and inflamed nerves. I don't blame the therapist; after all, I insisted on applying a lot of pressure, and neither of us was aware of my ongoing cervical condition.

Chapter 3

Initial Diagnosis

The light bulb in my head finally went off after years of agony. When I finally accepted that my constant and increasing pain was not from normal daily stress or overuse, I sought out help from my primary care physician (PCP). I wasn't only experiencing radiating pain, numbness and tingling in my right arm and shoulder; I was also experiencing myelopathy with neurological and muscle impairment. "Myelopathy" is any neurological deficit to the spinal cord, and in my case this meant compression of the spinal cord in the cervical area of the neck between levels C6 and C7. This was causing the neurological impairment and partial paralysis in my right hand and arm.

When the spinal cord is compressed, the electrical signals and messages being carried throughout the affected peripheral nerves are interrupted, and this can cause all sorts of neurological-related issues, as well as pain. The symptoms of myelopathy can come on subtly and get progressively worse over time, or be acute in nature. Becoming aware of these symptoms can help you identify them earlier and describe them more specifically to your physician.

Based on my medical history and description of pain (radiating right side neck and shoulder pain—known as "cervical radiculopathy"—coupled with numbness and tingling of my right thumb and middle fingers)—my primary care doctor suspected nerve impingement or injury of some sort at the C6-C7 level. He also didn't rule out other possible causes which could create similar symptoms, such as a tumor or cyst. In every case, symptoms such as these need further evaluation, so he referred me to a local orthopedic surgeon who specialized in spine and cervical issues.

Easing the Pain Between Appointments

To help manage the severe pain until my next appointment, my primary care physician (PCP) prescribed hydrocodone, prednisone and gabapentin. Gabapentin is an anticonvulsant used primarily to treat seizures and neuropathic pain, and in my case, it was prescribed to help relieve my neuropathic pain and allow me to sleep. Prednisone is a steroid, and was given to me to treat tissue and nerve inflammation. Anyone experiencing nerve pain at this level usually doesn't sleep well. And if you're reading this and know someone who is experiencing nerve-related pain due to neuropathy, do not underestimate how painful and debilitating this condition is. The pain is annoying and constant, causing discomfort, stress and agitation. In my case it was all-consuming and had infiltrated every aspect of my life. I couldn't really escape it.

Specialist Referral

My PCP referred me to a local, board-certified orthopedic spine surgeon. My appointment was scheduled the same week. Upon my visit to the surgeon's office, staff gathered the same historical medical information and biographical data that I'd shared with my PCP, and they quickly came to a similar impression that my pain was the result of nerve impingement and compression at the C6-C7 level.

The orthopedic surgeon ordered X-rays and an MRI. Although the X-rays confirmed some abnormality within the disc space of the spine, the MRI confirmed in great detail the exact cause of my nerve impingement.

Along with the detailed images that the MRI provided I also received a report generated by a radiologist (a physician specializing in interpreting X-rays, MRI's, CT scans and other diagnostic images). Although the MRI interpretation report I am sharing here was taken from my post-op follow-up *after* my ACDF surgery, I am sharing it at this point in my story to help familiarize you with what a radiologist's MRI interpretation report looks like. (The MRI report from my pre-ACDF diagnosis was unavailable for this book.)

The first report below is a copy of the unedited version (excluding my personal biographical data and information). The one that follows it defines some of the unfamiliar medical terminology and language. Although portions of the material do not lend themselves to simplification, I hope my explanations still clarify much of the report and assist you in becoming an informed patient.

Of course, your MRI results will vary, and some of the specific interpretive language on your report may differ from what was used on mine. So remember that if you have any questions regarding your MRI or X-ray report, do not hesitate to speak with the radiologist or your physician to help interpret and understand it.

My Actual Diagnostic Radiology Image Report
**Magnetic Resonance Imaging
Radiology Report**
Diagnostic Radiology Image Report **MRI**

PATIENT: Patrick Smith **DOB:** XXXXX

MRN: 123456

REFERING MD: XXXXXX

EXAM DATE: 01/01/2014

PROCEDURE: MRI CERVICAL SPINE

HISTORY:
Neck pain. Anterior spinal fusion in 2013.
COMPARISON:
None.
TECHNIQUE:
Multisequence multiplanar imaging obtained of the cervical spine using a 3 Tesla magnet.
FINDINGS:

The craniovertebral junction is unremarkable. Artifactual increased T2 signal is seen within the spinal cord on sagittal T2 sequence. The spinal cord is normal in morphology. Normal vascular flow voids are seen. 2 low signal intensity foci are seen within the left thyroid gland, likely calcification.

The vertebral body heights are maintained. The marrow is normal in signal intensity. There is sequela of anterior discectomy and fusion spanning C6-C7 and C7 transplant screws and intravertebral graft.

The skull base-C1 and C1-C2 facet articulations are intact.

C2-C3: The spinal canal and neural foramina are patent.

C3-C4: Minimal uncovertebral hypertrophy. Mild right and no left neural foraminal narrowing. Spinal canal is patent.

C4-C5: Small central disc protrusion minimally effacing the ventral thecal sac. Minimal uncovertebral hypertrophy causing minimal right neural foraminal narrowing. Left neural foramen is patent. Spinal canal is patent.

C5-C6: Right paracentral disc protrusion and annular fissure effacing the right ventral spinal canal. No Neural foraminal narrowing. There is mild bilateral uncovertebral hypertrophy causing mild bilateral neural foraminal narrowing.

C6-C7: Spinal canal and neural foramina are patent.

C7-T1: Central disc protrusion with a small annular fissure mildly effacing the ventral thecal sac. Spinal canal and neural foramina are patent. Straightening of the cervical lordosis.

IMPRESSION:
Sequela discectomy and anterior fusion spanning C6-C7 without hardware-related complication by MRI. Straightening of the cervical lordosis, either positional or related to muscle spasms.

Mild multilevel degenerative disc disease, greatest at C5-6 and C7-T1 without spinal canal stenosis.

Uncovertebral hypertrophy causes minimal to mild multilevel neural foraminal narrowing, greatest on the right at C3-C4 and bilaterally at C5-C6.

What follows below is the report with additional definitions to help translate it into layperson's terms. In general I have only defined a term in [ ] brackets at its first appearance in the report. As noted above, your own MRI results may be expressed in a different way and it will be important to discuss them with your physician. I simply hope that in sharing my own MRI report and "translation" with you, I can contribute to your greater understanding on your own journey to becoming an informed patient.

3: Initial Diagnosis

My Actual Diagnostic Radiology Image Report
(expounded in laymen's terms)

**Magnetic Resonance Imaging
Radiology Report
MRI**

PATIENT: Patrick Smith DOB: XXXXX
MRN: 123456
REFERING MD: XXXXXX
EXAM DATE: 01/01/2014
PROCEDURE: MRI CERVICAL SPINE

HISTORY:
Neck pain. Anterior [front] spinal [spine] fusion [joining and fusing two vertebrae together] in 2013 [this refers to my completed ACDF surgery]
COMPARISON:
None.
TECHNIQUE:
Multisequence multiplanar imaging [a data processing technique used to help create a more informative image] obtained of the cervical spine [neck] using a 3 Tesla magnet [a type of MRI scanner]
FINDINGS:
The craniovertebral junction [abbreviated as CVJ; this is a collective term that refers to the posterior/back/occiput of the skull base and supporting ligaments] is unremarkable [normal]. Artifactual increased T2 signal is seen within the spinal cord on sagittal [left and right halves] T2 sequence [this sentence describes a part of the technical process of the MRI, which uses a magnetic field to stimulate proton activity, generating signals that are converted by computer software into the pictures that are interpreted by your physician and radiologist.] The spinal cord is normal in morphology [the shape and structure of the spinal cord are normal]. Normal vascular flow voids are seen [blood flow in the area appears to be normal]. 2 low signal intensity foci [points of interest] are seen within the left thyroid gland, likely calcification [accumulation of calcium].

The vertebral body [a portion of the vertebra at the front of the spine] heights are maintained [the space between the vertebrae are even]. The marrow is normal in signal intensity [the bone marrow is normal]. There is sequela [condition related to previous disease or injury] of anterior discectomy and fusion spanning C6-C7 and C7 transplant screws and intravertebral graft [in other words, the fact that I had ACDF surgery is obvious from the images on the MRI].

The skull base-C1 and C1-C2 facet articulations [the joints in the spine are called "facets," and "articulations" refers to parts of one vertebra that connect it to another vertebra] are intact [not damaged or impaired].

C2-C3: The spinal canal and neural foramina [openings for nerve roots in the spinal canal] are patent [normal and unobstructed].

C3-C4: Minimal uncovertebral hypertrophy [enlargement of small synovial joints connecting two bones]. Mild right and no left neural foraminal narrowing [there is some small amount of narrowing of the openings for nerves in the spinal canal on the right, but not on the left side]. Spinal canal is patent [normal].

C4-C5: Small central disc protrusion [bulging; that is, the disc is pushing out of where it normally is] minimally effacing [compressing] the ventral [front] thecal sac [membrane that surrounds the spinal cord]. Minimal uncovertebral hypertrophy causing minimal right neural foraminal narrowing. Left neural foramen is patent. Spinal canal is patent.

C5-C6: Right paracentral disc protrusion and annular fissure [damage/tear] effacing the right ventral spinal canal. No Neural foraminal narrowing. There is mild bilateral uncovertebral hypertrophy causing mild bilateral neural foraminal narrowing.

C6-C7: Spinal canal and neural foramina are patent.

C7-T1: Central disc protrusion with a small annular fissure mildly effacing the ventral thecal sac. Spinal canal and neural foramina are patent. Straightening of the cervical lordosis [in my case, the spine is straight when it should be curved, although in general "lordosis" means that the spine is not curving the way it should, so it could refer to too great or too small a curve, or a curve in the wrong direction].

IMPRESSION:

Sequela discectomy and anterior fusion spanning C6-C7 without hardware-related complication by MRI. [The impression is that my condition is the result of a previous disease or injury and that

3: Initial Diagnosis

surgical removal of all or part of an intervertebral disc has taken place, as has a fusion of the front part of the vertebra spanning C6-C7, without any resulting complications involved with the hardware use to accomplish the fusion. In other words, I had ACDF surgery.] Straightening of the cervical lordosis either positional or related to muscle spasms.

Mild multilevel degenerative disc disease, greatest at C5-6 and C7-T1 without spinal canal stenosis [compression].

Uncovertebral hypertrophy causes minimal to mild multilevel neural foraminal narrowing, greatest on the right at C3-C4 and bilaterally at C5-C6.

As you can see from the radiologist's report and findings, my cervical spine has a number of complex issues going on which periodically cause pain and muscle spasms. If you have only one segment of disc that needs to be repaired with a partial discectomy or ACDF surgery, consider yourself lucky.

Problems with Diagnostic Testing

Sometimes patients, including myself, tend to want hard, concrete evidence to prove that their symptoms and condition are real. Medical testing and diagnostic imaging, like MRIs and X-rays, assist us on the path to confirmation and proper diagnosis. But this isn't always a good thing. Why not? We sometimes set ourselves up for failure by looking for evidence that proves the pain we're experiencing is caused by the defect we're seeing on the image. This phenomenon is known as "confirmation bias," which is "the tendency to search for, interpret, favor, and recall information in a way that confirms one's preexisting beliefs or hypotheses, while giving disproportionately less consideration to alternative possibilities." [4]

The evidence provided by MRIs, X-rays, and other testing methodologies does not always definitively indicate the source of the problem or pain you are experiencing. Confirmation bias can lead to another phenomenon once the evidence is presented to you: belief perseverance. Belief perseverance refers to a situation in which beliefs continue even after evidence that contradicts them is provided.

The takeaway is that diagnostic testing, including diagnostic imaging, is simply another tool that assists the physician in making an informed diagnosis in conjunction with the patient's symptoms. It does not always provide a definitive answer in and of itself, and your treatment team will usually consider it in conjunction with other

---

[4] Plous, Scott (1993). The Psychology of Judgment and Decision Making. p. 233.

elements of your medical history.

The Role of the Radiologist

Even though most physicians can get a general impression from MRI images, they are typically not specifically trained for such detailed interpretations unless they are radiologists. A radiologist's report and MRI make up an extremely important part of the process to help the physician and/or surgeon make the proper diagnosis and assist with the surgery itself. Without this detailed report the surgeon would not be able to confirm his initial impression to help make a proper diagnosis. Consequently, having an experienced radiologist provide a written report is a critical component of the overall diagnostic process and surgery.

In my own case, after my MRI I was scheduled for a follow-up appointment later in the week.

Chapter 4

Surgical Consultation

The Choice of a Surgeon

Although I had already been to an orthopedic surgeon's office for my MRI and was scheduled to follow up with that doctor, I researched several other orthopedic and neurospine surgeons who specialized in cervical and spinal fusions. It just made sense to me to gather information about the different options and approaches that were available to me. I would have done the same thing if I were going to make any major decision that would affect my life, and ACDF surgery seemed like such a decision to me.

My informal research took the form of conversations with doctors, friends and acquaintances in the medical field, as well as patient comments and reviews on websites related to cervical spine surgery. The information I gathered made me aware that I had a range of options.

I had friends who worked in the local medical field, including an acquaintance who was an orthopedic surgeon. He advised me to look for information about general surgical issues, average infection rates, complications, and other mitigating factors involved in complicated surgeries, such as cervical fusion surgery.

In some respects, it would've been easier to just go ahead with the surgery without the additional complications of researching surgeons and related issues. But in this case doing my due diligence was a valuable part of my process of becoming an informed patient, and it may have prevented an unwanted outcome.

My First Surgical Consultation

The week after my MRI I met with the orthopedic surgeon who was initially recommended to do my surgery. The appointment was for a follow-up and surgical consultation. He reviewed my MRI report and images with me. As suspected there was disc protrusion (bulging disc) at the C6-C7 level against my spinal cord, as well as disc protrusions at the C4-C5 and C5-C6 levels, though these were not as severe in general; specifically, they did not present with acute nerve impingement and motor deficit, and I had no symptomatic pain from them. The surgeon recommended that I have a multilevel fusion of the three discs in question. That surgical option would have fused three vertebrae together with one plate—greatly limiting my neck mobility.

This was the first time I really confronted the idea that I needed ACDF surgery. Up to that point the thought of surgery had not quite sunk in, and I simply didn't know what to expect. I felt a bit shocked after hearing the surgeon's evaluation of my symptoms and condition, as well as his radical approach and recommendation to undergo a multi-level fusion. As he explained the medical procedure and instrumentation that would be used during the operation, I couldn't help but think, "Isn't this a bit too aggressive?" I found the surgeon to be professional, but I wondered if everything he was recommending was absolutely necessary. (Obviously different surgeons will have different opinions.) When the consultation was over, something did not sit well with me. I felt pressured and uneasy.

Seeking a Second Opinion

After the consultation I realized I had a lot of investigating to do

4: Surgical Consultation

about ACDF surgery and whether there were other options available to me. I immediately began seeking a second opinion. At the time, I wasn't concerned about the safety of the surgery itself; I was more concerned about the best approach to it, and about who would be conducting it.

I asked some of my family and friends for recommendations. This included a friend who is an orthopedic foot and ankle surgeon. I had always respected him and valued his thoughts. He also encouraged me to seek out a second opinion, and recommended another surgeon, Dr. Mark Davidson.[5] He said that if he or his family needed neck or back surgery, he would want Dr. Davidson to perform it. In my friend's view, surgeons are more like artists, and I didn't necessarily need to travel to a big city to find a great surgeon. Some surgeons prefer to work for themselves and often open their own private practice. This allows them to be in control of their own practice rather than being inundated with the kind of administrative bureaucracy and policy they are more likely to encounter at a group practice or hospital.

That was what I needed to hear. I began to feel a bit of relief, because the process of choosing a surgeon had become a bit overwhelming.

Neurosurgeon or Orthopedic Surgeon?

I also considered seeking out the consultation of a neurosurgeon who specialized in spine surgery, although in the end I thought it best to find a talented orthopedic surgeon. Although neurosurgeons are just as capable of performing ACDF surgery, I didn't think it was necessary. In my opinion, and for my own individual situation, it came down to individual performance, talent and surgical history, as

---

[5] Names and identifying details have been changed.

well as how many ACDF surgeries the physician had successfully performed. Based on the research I did and articles I read on the topic, it was my opinion that ACDF surgery was more of a mechanical and structural surgery that didn't involve manipulation of any small nerves or microsurgery. It also seemed that more often it was orthopedic surgeons specializing in spine surgery who performed ACDF surgeries. I simply felt more comfortable seeking out a talented and reputable board-certified orthopedic spine surgeon.

ACDF surgery does not typically require the delicate manipulation of nerves—unless there are complications. Although the surgery is performed only millimeters away from the spinal cord, it does not involve the direct manipulation of the spinal cord or surrounding nerves.

My thoughts and opinions aside, one can argue the case either way for which type of surgeon to use, and both types of surgeons are just as capable.

I wanted a surgeon who had years of experience conducting successful ACDF surgeries with the least amount of patient complications and complaints. I also understood that any surgery comes with certain risks, up to and including death. The most unexpected things can happen during surgery, even to the most talented of surgeons. This is why it's important to interview and ask your surgeon lots of questions related to your specific surgery.

That said, if my surgery was going to be complicated and involve microsurgery or the manipulation of the spinal cord or peripheral nerves, I would have sought out a neurosurgeon who specialized in conducting such procedures. If your diagnosis is complicated and involves multiple levels or the manipulation of nerves and related conditions, make sure you ask your surgeon if a neurosurgeon or specialist should be involved. If you don't feel comfortable with the answers you receive, consider seeking a second or third opinion. And as always, please remember that I am sharing my opinions and personal experiences in this book, and these are not a substitute for the medical advice of a physician. The material I outline here is intended to give you more information to discuss with your physician as part of your own decision-making process.

The Second Surgical Consultation

After making the decision to seek out a second opinion I scheduled an appointment with Dr. Davidson, the orthopedic surgeon recommended by my friend. Dr. Davidson carried all the necessary qualifications I was looking for and was board certified. During my consultation I immediately felt at ease and comforted. He was a down-to-earth, normal kind of guy who was not in any way offended by my questions. I could also tell he was confident and up-to-date with the most recent medical information and technology regarding ACDF surgery.

Probably the most important attribute he possessed, besides his surgical skills, was his work ethic and accountability to his patients. He told me he was trained in the ways of traditional medicine and surgical practices, all of which demanded long hours, and for good reason. He said that he didn't want to pass off his patients to other physicians who were not directly involved in their care. Dr. Davidson's approach to caregiving meant early starts to his days and longer hours, because he gave each patient comprehensive personal attention.

Why should this be important to you? Your surgeon's approach can directly impact your care. Today, many physicians specialize so much that they do not maintain a close patient relationship throughout the surgery; consequently, they are not as familiar with a patient's medical history. I believe that when they do this they are doing the patient a disservice. Many patients have complicated medical histories that can only be understood by a physician who has an intimate, personal patient-physician relationship. So while specialists are a necessary part of modern medicine, it's possible that the emphasis on referring patients to other physicians for follow-up has gone too far and can leave critical patient information out of the equation.

Questioning the Doctor

Dr. Davidson allowed me to ask anything I wanted to, and this included many of the typical questions a patient in my shoes might have, including how many ACDF procedures he had performed (he said he had lost count, but he believed he'd performed more than 1,100 ACDF surgeries to date).

He wasn't offended by my questions. I actually thought I was being an annoying patient, but he stated he was glad to see an informed patient asking the right questions. What I want to stress here is that you too might want to learn to ask the right questions and seek out a second opinion, especially if you do not feel comfortable with your surgeon. Let your intuition and conscience help you make the right choice. ACDF surgery is a big deal, and the outcome of the surgery can have long-lasting consequences. There are risks to any surgery—but you can at least try to mitigate those risks by asking the right questions.

Don't be shy: seek out the information you need and ask the important questions.

The Implant

After careful consideration Dr. Davidson recommended that I have one-level (C6-C7) ACDF surgery using the Medtronic Sofamor Danek USA, Inc., PEEK Prevail® system Medtronic Inc., PEEK Prevail® brand cervical interbody device. Following a more

4: Surgical Consultation

traditional approach and standard protocol for ACDF surgery, he stated he did not believe fusing the other two levels was necessary because the other discs were not causing neurological symptoms, motor deficit or impairment. He did warn me that I might need a second surgery in the future to repair the other levels if I began to develop neurological symptoms and pain, but he also stated that there was no telling how long the other discs might hold up. (At the time of this writing I'm on my eighth year post-operative without other cervical symptoms. I think I made the right choice. I'm hoping to go many more years without having to undergo another surgery.)

Dr. Davidson stated that although there were many different hardware and implant options on the market to choose from, he used the Medtronic Sofamor Danek Ltd., PEEK Prevail® system. He believed the PEEK Prevail® system was one of the most simple and reliable interbody devices and offered the best long-term patient outcome with the least complications. According to Medtronic's informational data, Medtronic conducted one of the largest long-term patient studies with respect to interbody cervical devices, studying more than 500 patients using the PEEK Prevail® system.[6]

I researched other devices and methods out of curiosity, and although some devices offered flexible systems and other types of hardware, their long-term reliability was unknown, and some had higher rates of post-operative complications. The information I found on other devices did not provide enough data with regard to long-term patient use, potential complications, and outcomes. I was not willing to become a test Guinea pig and risk my personal health and quality of life. I agreed with Dr. Davidson's choice of the PEEK Prevail® system interbody device.

(It's important to note here that I'm not personally endorsing the device for everyone. In fact, by the time you read this book there will

---

[6]http://www.gahpl.com/pdf/cervical/PEEK_PREVAIL_Surgical_Technique.pdf

likely be other more advanced products on the market, both from Medtronic and other companies. All I would like to point out here is that I did my research to make the best-informed decision I could at that time, and I suggest you do the same.)

The PEEK Prevail® system uses a chambered polyetheretherketone (a kind of high-tech, high-performance plastic) implant that serves as the replacement disc. The chambers of the PEEK disc are filled with the patient's own harvested bone, which is usually taken from the iliac crest (pelvis or hip). This autologous graft, or "autograft," when healed, is what holds and "fuses" the upper and lower vertebrae together. The hardware utilized during the operation supports the joint while the healing process takes place. Once healing is complete the vertebrae are fused together and are strong and stable. The hardware remains, although it is no longer needed to stabilize the joint.

Allograft

Another method utilized to fuse joints—in this case the cervical spine—is called "allograft." Allograft uses a donor bone, usually from a cadaver, which will grow together as the healing process takes place. Hardware is also used in this type of fusion to assist with the healing process. The possible complications with both types of cervical fusion procedures are that the bone graft or donor bone might fail to grow or be rejected, resulting in pseudarthrosis—also known as a false joint or non-union.

Dr. Cole, Professor in the Departments of Orthopedic Surgery and Anatomy and Cell Biology at Rush University Medical Center, conducted a study with two hundred patients who had undergone ACDF surgery to determine post-operative fusion success rates. His study revealed that a single level allograft (fusion) had a 95% success

4: Surgical Consultation

rate after five years.[7] Those are pretty good statistics. Nonetheless, although my fusion was a success, I was mentally prepared to deal with the possibility of a failure and second surgery.

Maintaining a healthy body is important prior to surgery for many reasons, including reducing risk factors like pseudarthrosis. Smoking, obesity, alcohol and a sedentary lifestyle, for example, all increase the risk of surgery and failed fusions as well as other complications.

During my surgical consultation, Dr. Davidson explained the usual protocols he engaged in prior to and during surgery. He let me know that he had a "clean room" agreement with the hospital where the surgery was being performed. This meant that the day prior to the surgery, Dr. Davidson's staff personally cleaned and disinfected the operating room and all equipment. The room was sealed off after it was cleaned, and was not opened again until the day of surgery. This was an important fact that I had overlooked during my research process. The possibility of an infection during surgery at any medical institution is a real concern. I appreciated the surgeon going the extra mile for his patients' care. In reality it shouldn't be any other way.

Dr. Davidson explained that he didn't want to wait too long to do the surgery because the myelopathy and neuropathy I was experiencing could become permanent if left untreated. From what I had already learned during my research, I knew this to be true. Nerve compression left untreated can cause long-term nerve damage and related effects. I really didn't feel like I had an option. I scheduled the surgery approximately two weeks out from my consultation. Dr. Davidson's staff provided me with the patient information I needed for the upcoming surgery and assisted me with the appropriate

---

[7] Hofheinz, Elizabeth. "General Topics Feature." Orthopedics This Week, 24 Feb. 2014, ryortho.com/2014/02/new-study-95-meniscal-allograft-survival-rate-acdf-non-fusion-rate-higher-than-expected-are-antibiotic-containing-balls-the-future-of-infection-prevention/

insurance paperwork and approvals.

I personally feel that Dr. Davidson was an exceptional choice for me. With that said, your choice of physician is *your* choice, and I strongly encourage you to do your own research on *any* physician whom you're considering for your care. This includes understanding their policies and procedures and those of their overall practice. And the more research you've done on your injury or condition, the better off you will be evaluating the surgeon's qualifications and specialties. It's all part of being an informed patient.

Before Surgery and Pre-Operative Consultation

Two weeks prior to surgery I eliminated all unhealthy food (including alcohol) and began eating healthy superfoods. I'd also stepped up my intake of fruits, vegetables, and essential vitamins to supplement my diet. Luckily, I was in fairly good physical shape prior to surgery, which helped during the recovery process post-op.

Your pre-operative instructions may vary according to your age, health, current medical condition, and medications. If I had known earlier that I would be undergoing ACDF surgery I would have been even better prepared physically. One of the benefits of a rapid onset of symptoms followed up by surgery is that you don't have much time to overthink the process or worry. Although not everyone can help their current medical condition, I think everyone should try to put their health first prior to surgery, which helps reduce the chances of complications and increase the chances of a speedier recovery.

Blood Testing

Approximately two weeks prior to surgery I met with Dr. Davidson to ask any final questions I might have, and also so he could give me pre-operative instructions. He directed me to have my blood drawn for testing, a common practice even for healthy patients

4: Surgical Consultation

prior to surgery. The blood panel tests performed before surgery usually include a full blood panel, CBC (Complete Blood Count), WBC (White Blood Count), and glucose, potassium, and coagulation study tests, among other things, to ensure patients aren't anemic and that they don't have other issues which might pose a risk during surgery. Blood tests tell the physician if a patient is healthy enough to undergo surgery and can reveal other illnesses which might complicate the surgery. More testing may be requested if you have special circumstances or other health issues.

Anesthesiologist

Prior to my surgery I also met with the anesthesiologist, who is another important medical figure in any surgical procedure. My anesthesiologist had a working agreement with Dr. Davidson and performed with him during most of his surgical procedures. He conducted a personal interview, asking me questions that pertained to anything that might interfere with his ability to successfully perform full-body (or "general") anesthesia. Full-body anesthesia is a chemically induced state of deep sleep in which the patient is not consciously aware of pain. Some of the questions the anesthesiologist asked included ones about my current overall health, medications and medical history.

The anesthesiologist also checked my mouth and airway and tested my gag reflex. These checks are performed to ensure the patient maintains an open airway during intubation. An intubation device, called an endotracheal tube (ET), is used to keep the patient's airway open and to deliver oxygen during the surgical procedure. During my interview with the anesthesiologist he noticed I was nervous about the operation and suggested I take diazepam—generic Valium—the night before surgery, if needed, and the morning of the operation to help calm any anxiety I might have prior to surgery.

Diazepam also has what I considered a beneficial side effect in this context: amnesic syndrome (or simply "amnesia"). In other words, it can cause the patient to have both short-term and long-term memory loss. The anesthesiologist told me that this amnesic effect might help reduce psychological stress throughout the surgical process. Note that diazepam and its related family of drugs (benzodiazepenes) are prescription-only and are potentially addictive, so the normal precautions regarding their use apply, and they should only be used as necessary and under the guidance of your physician.

Neither Dr. Davidson nor the anesthesiologist found any health-related concerns prior to my surgery, and I was given a clean bill of health.

Chapter 5

Surgery and Post-Op

I was given instructions not to eat or drink after 6:00 p.m. the night before surgery, and to wash myself with antimicrobial soap both that evening and the next morning (standard protocol for most surgeries).

NPO is an acronym for the Latin term *nil per os*, meaning "nothing by mouth." Most hospitals and medical facilities have protocols in place that state patients undergoing surgery should refrain from eating or drinking eight to twelve hours prior to surgery, and this was the recommendation for me. This policy was primarily put in place to reduce the chance of pulmonary aspiration during surgery. Under general anesthesia your normal swallowing and gag reflexes don't work. You are also likely to have an endotracheal tube in place, which is a tube placed down the throat to keep you breathing, so if food should rise up from your stomach your gag reflex will not function to clear your airway.

As the night before my surgery dragged on, I couldn't help but begin to think about all the possible negative outcomes: death, paralysis, and so on. Then I remembered that the anesthesiologist had prescribed me diazepam to help with anxiety and restless sleep, both of which can be common psychological responses prior to surgery. I knew getting a good night's sleep was an essential part of putting my body in the best place health-wise prior to surgery, so I took my prescribed diazepam.

I woke up early the morning of surgery, got ready and headed out the door with my wife, who drove me to the hospital. Prior to arriving at the hospital, I again took diazepam to calm my nerves, as I knew I would be anxious.

I was glad to have my wife drive me; even if I hadn't taken diazepam —which would have interfered with my driving—it made sense not to drive myself. It was not only the safe thing to do, it was the right thing to do. I wouldn't be in any condition to drive after surgery and so would need to arrange for someone else to drive me home anyway. Besides, anyone can be arrested for driving while impaired or under the influence of prescription medication. All surgeons will most certainly require patients have a driver after surgery. Usually a patient undergoing ACDF surgery will have one overnight stay at the hospital and not be released the same day. This protocol is in place so the patient can be monitored for potential post-operative complications.

After arriving at the hospital for check-in and registration, which I can hardly remember due to diazepam's amnesic effects, I was interviewed again by the attending nurse and anesthesiologist. As a precaution to ensure proper medical care is given to the patient, pre-screening questions prior to surgery are a normal part of the process. I have only a vague memory of being wheeled into the operating room and administered anesthesia prior to surgery.

Post-operative Recovery

And then, just like that—it seemed—I was done. My most recent memory after surgery is of being in the hospital room. This is not to be confused with the "recovery" room or step-down unit where a patient is brought immediately after surgery. After officially "waking up" and regaining consciousness and a greater awareness of my surroundings, I realized I was uncomfortable, stiff, and in a bit of pain—but the acute radiating nerve pain in my neck and arm were gone. The discomfort and pain I was feeling were from the surgery itself and are very common.

Other than the post-op pain and dysphasia (which I will discuss below), the surgery was a complete success.

I was thirsty and requested water with ice as my throat was sore and swollen from the incision and being intubated. I learned that after the operation I had been brought into the surgery step-down unit, also known as a post-anesthesia care unit (PACU), where patients are monitored until the effects of the anesthesia wear off and consciousness is regained. I didn't remember being in the step-down unit after the surgery, and most patients do not.

Dysphasia

I mentioned above that I was experiencing post-op dysphasia. Dysphasia is difficulty swallowing, and it's very common after ACDF surgery. No one had told me about this phenomenon. Although its pathophysiology is unclear, most ACDF patients will experience some form of dysphasia immediately after surgery. Although it usually goes away over time, dysphasia can continue for several days, weeks, months or even years. It can even become a permanent condition after ACDF surgery, but this is very rare. Usually symptoms only last a few weeks.

I personally experienced moderate dysphasia for weeks after the surgery, and mild dysphasia for months. This condition slowly got better, though I still experienced mild symptoms of dysphasia for three years post-op. The brain has a way of ignoring mild irritations via selective filtering, so it wasn't much of a problem for me. Only on occasion did I notice it.

In any case, expect some form of dysphasia and difficulty swallowing immediately after ACDF surgery.

Pain

I requested pain medication once the effects of anesthesia wore off and the pain began to settle in. I was given morphine sulfate, approximately .05–0.1 mg/kg (intravenous—IV) about every 2-4 hours to assist with pain management. Growing up I thought that morphine was the most powerful pain medication on the planet. I figured if the nurses were administering it to me it must be for good reason. I soon realized that morphine was not particularly strong with respects to post-op ACDF surgery pain, and that its effects are to some extent dependent on the person and their personal pain threshold and physiology, as well as other factors. I've since learned that morphine is in the low to mid-range scale with respects to pain medication.

I underestimated the amount of pain I would experience after surgery. A few hours post-op I realized that morphine wasn't cutting it. I asked the nurses if there was something else besides morphine in the spectrum of pain medication that could be given.

In my experience, nurses tend to get annoyed if patients keep asking for pain medication, but when you're in pain you just want relief. On the other hand, I think most physicians and nurses know that patients undergoing surgery are in pain and have likely been taking pain medication prior to surgery. They also understand that tolerance builds quickly and that the longer a patient has been on pain medication, the stronger their medication may need to be to manage post-op pain. Ultimately, giving patients only the amount of pain medication necessary to stop the pain is the goal, and this can take some figuring out post-op.

As the evening progressed I struggled to sleep. It seemed that no matter what position I adopted in bed, it was uncomfortable. The feeling was akin to being hit by a truck. With the approval of my doctor I was administered the pain medication Demerol, an opiate generically known as meperidine. I suspect that my tolerance to opioid-based medication had built up prior to surgery, which only takes a few days to occur. I had been prescribed hydrocodone two weeks earlier to combat the pain I had been experiencing from neuropathy.

After the Demerol was administered I was able to fall asleep.

The Day After

The morning of my discharge I woke up about 4:00 a.m. Waking up after ACDF surgery was a bit daunting. I had to do a little self-therapy to get myself going—basically focusing my willpower to get out of bed. I didn't want to get up, but I obviously had to, and it wasn't going to happen all by itself. I was groggy, and as I slowly got moving and dressed I tried to distract myself from the aching, dull pain by listening to the nurses go about their business checking on patients.

When I finally got up and mobile, I started snooping around on a quest for coffee. The nurses were kind enough to give me a cup of their personal brew. If patients are rude, bark orders and complain, nurses won't go out of their way to assist them. I would personally recommend suffering in silence and only calling them when needed (but *do* call on them when needed). Remember, you're not the only patient. And it's one thing to actually need assistance for something; it's another to complain or be dismissive simply because you're experiencing normal post-surgery discomfort. Even if you're in pain and need help, try to remember to be nice to the nurses; it's simple courtesy, and it will also pay off during your stay.

My doctor arrived at 6:00 a.m. to make his rounds. He was surprised to see me up and about. I was ready to go home and sleep in my own bed. He explained that even though I had just had surgery and felt like I couldn't move my neck, the mechanical structure of the joint was intact and stable, and movement was not limited. He said most of my perceived limitations were psychosomatic. Most of the pain I was experiencing from the surgery was from the small, lateral 1½-inch incision in the front of my neck. When a surgeon makes the first incision for ACDF surgery they enter from the front (anterior) of the neck and pierce the outer layer of skin (called the epidermis), and then move into the dermis. Once the initial incision is performed, a second, smaller, vertical incision is made through a band of muscle tissue on the lower side of the neck just above the collar bone. I think a majority of the pain comes from cutting into the thin layer of muscle tissue.

Keep in mind that I had other ongoing issues which were also causing pain.[8] If you're one of the lucky few who recover quickly without complications and severe pain, more power to you. However, if you have other health-related issues on top of cervical ones, you may want to consider managing and compartmentalizing each issue separately so as not to become overwhelmed. Sometimes compartmentalizing each ailment and overcoming each one separately helps manage and reduce psychological stress. Some patients underestimate the challenges of the recovery process and the length of time it can take to recover; I know I did. Finding a balanced solution and managing each health issue using many different modalities is key.

Prior to being discharged from the hospital, my doctor prescribed hydrocodone to help me manage the pain while recovering. Although the acute nerve pain I'd been experiencing prior to surgery subsided, the pain from the surgery—coupled with an insidious new type of

---

[8] These included a torn ACL on my right knee, a broken back (also known as a "Scotty Dog" fracture) from an unknown injury, arthritis and assorted other injuries resulting from past accidents.

post-op pain—set in. We'll explore this common challenge in the next chapter, "Understanding and Managing Pain."

Neck Brace

My doctor explained that not only did I not need a neck brace, he had found that neck braces hinder recovery time and give the patient a false sense of security. He told me to take it easy—I might feel like I could do a lot physically, but I shouldn't overdo it. For the most part I wasn't limited physically from moving my head from side to side or up and down. As I've already mentioned, he explained that most of the limitations I felt were psychosomatic, probably due to my brain telling my body that I'd had surgery and sending out pain signals.

These days, after having fully recovered, and having talked with other patients who've undergone ACDF surgery and worn cervical braces, I would agree with my doctor that recovery seems to be faster without the brace. I also feel that not wearing the cervical brace and keeping my neck in motion reduced pain. I know that other orthopedic surgeons prefer patients to wear a neck brace after ACDF surgery. There may be other reasons that help a surgeon determine which patients they want wearing a cervical brace. So, needless to say, talk with your doctor about this issue. In my own case, in hindsight, I think my doctor didn't want to make a big deal out of the situation, and in his opinion I wasn't a candidate for a brace.

So he shook my hand and said, "I'll see you in two weeks for a follow-up visit."

Going Home

Most ACDF surgeries are now considered outpatient ambulatory surgery. This protocol was changed years earlier based on pressure from health insurance carriers due to escalating healthcare costs. Keeping patients overnight or long-term in a hospital or other medical facility is very expensive. A one-night stay, or sometimes even being released the same day after a surgical procedure, is common nowadays.

After being discharged from the hospital, I was driven home by my wife, and my road to recovery began. What I didn't realize when I first set foot on this road was how long it would take. In fact, it took more than three years to find a balanced solution to manage the mild pain I experienced post-op. But again, I had other cervical issues going on so this may not be the case for you. I imagine that, without my other medical conditions, my full recovery time would have been reduced to about a year. I'd gone into this surgery having done a lot of research, but not nearly enough, especially about post-op recovery. I found out afterwards that I'd sorely underestimated how long the recovery process would take and just how painful it would be.

I have often wondered what would have been better: not knowing about the procedure and the subsequent pain and recovery, or having full knowledge of what was to be expected. I feel comfortable saying that being informed and aware of what was to be expected was the better choice, and if I could have been even *more* prepared, that would have been ideal. I think preparing mentally kept me from doing more harm to myself with respect to managing pain and overdoing it physically. I believe going blindly into surgery sets a patient up for additional challenges and unrealistic expectations.

Recovery

For the most part the recovery process was slow and painful. I didn't have a difficult time moving around, walking or doing everyday activities, but I did have trouble sleeping. The pain made it difficult to get comfortable, and I tossed and turned most nights for several months after surgery. Looking back now, I realize there were mini-milestones throughout the recovery process that blended into each other. In hindsight I should have requested some sort of benzodiazipine, an anti-anxiety and muscle relaxant medication, or discussed this more with my physician to help manage pain and sleep issues.

For the first three weeks following surgery the pain signals just kept on coming, and the only way I could manage the pain was with the assistance of pain and anticonvulsant medication to help keep me asleep. Sleep deprivation heightened my pain perception, and this became a vicious cycle.

The pain medication worked so well that when I had taken it, I forgot I'd even had surgery and felt normal. But this is a dangerous game to play because you can start to rely too much on the medicine. Of course, after the pain medication wore off the pain inevitably returned, so over a period of approximately two months, as things slowly got better I tapered off my pain medication.

I eventually substituted my prescription pain medication with acetaminophen and ibuprofen, both of which are over-the-counter pain medications. (Again, always discuss any changes you want to make with your physician.)

I will discuss pain management in greater depth in the next two chapters. For now I'll just say that it took about four to six months post-op before I felt able to begin exercising and running at a reasonable level. Atrophy of my muscles and general malaise had set in quickly during the sedentary recovery process. I tried to stretch and move around as much as possible. Stagnation is terrible for the body and health in general. I ate healthy and took vitamin supplements to speed the recovery process. I took hot showers and constantly sought out massages of my shoulder and neck as they became extremely fatigued and tense. It took approximately one year post-op to where I felt I was back to "normal."

All that said, in my opinion, and in the absence of other complications or health issues, the likelihood of a full recovery from one-level ACDF surgery is very good. Looking back, I am extremely grateful to my surgeon for his professionalism and care; essentially, he gave me my life back.

Chapter 6

Understanding and Managing Pain

The Nature of Pain

Although it may seem easy to define in relative terms, pain is a mysterious and complex phenomena in its pathophysiology. It is generally described as "a distressing feeling often caused by intense or damaging stimuli."[9] Nonetheless, the phenomena of pain can be a difficult concept to pin down. As individuals, we know when we're in pain, and we know that pain is an uncomfortable psychological experience. But pain has many different meanings to many different people and everyone has their own pain threshold.

I have come to believe that people who are constantly bombarded with pain signals become overly sensitive to them. In fact, they become hypersensitive. This phenomenon is called hyperalgesia, and patients experiencing it are susceptible to several health-related symptoms, including a heightened state of pain, depression and anxiety.

For the purposes of our discussion here it might be useful to touch on some of the different types of pain. For example, pain can be acute or chronic, and people can experience "nociceptive" and

---

[9] "Pain." Wikipedia. October 23, 2020. Accessed October 28, 2020. https://en.wikipedia.org/wiki/Pain.

"neuropathic" pain. Nociceptive pain is usually caused by injury or inflammation, such as when you stub your toe, break a bone, or burn yourself. Neuropathic pain, generally speaking, is caused by damage to the nervous system, and can also be acute or chronic.

This is hardly an exhaustive discussion, but it is useful to understand the overall basic concept and physiology of pain as it relates to ACDF surgery so you can better understand which of the available treatment options may work for you.

Pain and the Informed Patient

Well-informed patients who understand the basic concepts of pain increase their odds of managing their own pain more effectively by being better able to communicate and articulate exactly how they are feeling—and, most importantly, by being able to better understand their pain. This can be of great assistance to physicians. What's more, not understanding the basic concepts of pain, pain management, and available treatment options is a slippery slope. Pain can directly impact a patient's quality of life. Patients who are simply seeking an easy way out of pain may face detrimental health consequences involving the abuse of or addiction to potent prescription pain medications.

I began to really investigate and understand the phenomenon of pain only when I was experiencing it intensely and chronically myself. Luckily, I had a great, caring and intelligent primary care provider who not only understood pain but who also respected me as a patient. Over time we developed a trusting relationship; I trusted him, and he trusted me. He knew I had a great fear of the dangers of pain medication and that I struggled to seek relief without becoming dependent on medication.

In addition to mainstream medicine, I've also tried to manage my pain using alternative and natural approaches, some of which I will

6: Understanding and Managing Pain

discuss below. These methods are not always accepted by mainstream healthcare providers, but I was open to a variety of options for alleviating pain, and I knew I could always return to more traditional methods as needed.

Post-op ACDF Adjustment-Phase Pain

From my own experience, and from the experiences of others with whom I've spoken to who have had ACDF surgery, everyone must overcome and learn to live with post-op ACDF-related pain. This is the pain most ACDF patients experience that no one tells you about.

I call this type of pain "post-op ACDF adjustment-phase pain." Post-surgery is when the body begins to adjust to its new physiological state based on the surgical changes it has undergone. It is essentially creating a "new normal" for itself as it heals. I believe this post-op adjustment-phase pain arises from multiple sources, including physical, psychological, and pathophysiological ones. These can correlate to the muscular system, nervous system and fascia.

There are many effective ways to manage the related symptoms of post-op ACDF pain. For example, there are many prescription and over-the-counter products to choose from, as well as nutritional supplements. It has taken me many years of experimenting with physical therapy, exercise, yoga, meditation, acupuncture, nutrition, and prescription and OTC medications to help me manage my pain in a safe manner. Working with your PCP or PMP to figure out what works for you is the safest method.

In my own case, many of the different types of OTC and natural alternative supplements, medicines, treatments and modalities I tried did not work for me. Ultimately I found that a comprehensive approach—which included lots of physical exercise to manage my post-op ACDF related pain—worked, and continues to work, best for me in conjunction with other simple and effective treatments.

If you're reading this and are feeling anxious or depressed about your current condition, remember that things will get better with time. I hope that this book will be able to help you extract some useful information and concepts to support you along your journey.

Pain Scales

How does severe pain from cervical neuropathy rank in relation to other types of pain? To give you an indicator of my own pain I'll refer to the standard medical pain scale method, which usually uses a numerical scale of 1-10.

When I was initially diagnosed with cervical disc protrusion and neuropathy by my GP, and just prior to surgery, I was at a pain level of 7-8 out of 10, with 10 being excruciating and unbearable pain. Pain scales have a strong subjective element, since people experience pain differently, but I think that I have a fairly high degree of pain tolerance, and dealing with this type of acute pain is almost unbearable. I couldn't imagine living at this level of pain without the use of pain medication or other intervention. While writing this book I spoke with someone who admitted to me that he'd once thought about committing suicide to escape the pain he experienced after ACDF surgery and with some other ongoing medical issues. Thankfully he has since found healthy ways to manage his pain, but when it was as bad as it was, he felt like he was being "held captive" and controlled by his pain. If you are feeling this kind of pain yourself, know that it *can* get better—and don't hesitate to seek help from physicians and therapists. You don't have to do this alone.

Physician Choice: General Practitioner or Specialist?

Managing pain also includes having access to a knowledgeable and competent pain management physician or family physician.

6: Understanding and Managing Pain

Having a great, open relationship with an intelligent and caring primary care physician can be a big help when you're seeking relief from ACDF-related pain symptoms. When your doctor knows you, he or she is in a far better position to understand your particular needs, especially in the context of any other health issues you may have. He or she may also be easier to get an appointment with, and won't need to spend half of your appointment getting familiar with your case.

Specialists trained in pain management, on the other hand, are experts in their field. They may, for example, be more familiar with the latest treatment options and truly understand the phenomenon of pain intimately. They can be invaluable, especially for intractable problems. But wait times to see them can be extensive, they are often more expensive, and you may have to jump through additional hoops with your insurance company for approval to see them. Another factor is that, perhaps because of the national opioid crisis, some family physicians aren't comfortable with the administration, responsibility, and stigma associated with caring for patients with chronic or post-operative pain management. Your general practitioner may recommend that you see a specialist for this or any number of other reasons.

In my own personal experience, any competent and informed family medical physician or general practitioner is just as capable as a specialist in treating common ailments and general pain associated with ACDF surgery, including chronic pain conditions. Barring any specialty procedures such as ESI (epidural steroid injection), I've found that my family physician better understood my condition, and my care under him was unparalleled. As already mentioned, your family doctor is more likely to be familiar with your overall health. He or she may also have more time to spend with you than a specialist, although this is not always the case.

What is certainly true is that every individual has different needs, and over the course of your care you may try several different approaches yourself. I think my own doctor understood my moral compass as a patient and an ethical and responsible individual who was suffering. Even though he is inundated day-in and day-out with patients coming and going, he spends a good amount of time with everyone. He demonstrates the highest professionalism and standard of patient care and does so with compassion. If you can find a general practitioner who does the same, their guidance will be of immense support to you on your own journey.

Coping and Family Support

When someone suffers chronic pain, their loved ones are usually "co-sufferers." It's challenging to see someone you care about suffer. Also, side effects of chronic pain include irritability and frustration, and this can negatively impact relationships.

One of the challenges in this dynamic is that only you know exactly how you feel, and it can be difficult to convey this feeling to others. However, it's important to try. Communicating with your family or significant other about how you're feeling will greatly reduce misunderstandings and frustration. At the same time, try to accept that not everyone will be able to truly comprehend the experiences and pain you will go through as an ACDF patient, except perhaps another ACDF patient.

I would highly recommend that your significant other, partner, or a family member attend your pre-surgery and post-surgery appointments. Having a trusted third party attend these appointments not only boosts your sense of psychological support, it may also provide important insights and context. When others are present and hear the interactions between doctor and patient, it helps them see things from a different perspective and it opens a door of compassion, understanding and communication. Seeing just how frustrating and complicated managing pain is makes things easier for them to understand what you are going through.

In my own case, I learned very quickly that my wife did not want to listen to me constantly whine and complain about my pain. I had to accept that she would never fully understand—although she tried—and that it wasn't her responsibility to do so. Unfortunately, our loved ones can become victims of the ACDF pain management process as well. But raising our awareness of this issue helps mitigate it.

Chapter 7

Pain Management Modalities

Many Modalities: What Works for You?

I have mentioned this several times already, but it bears repeating: Everything I share in this book is simply my own experience and research. Under no circumstances should you experiment with any of the discussed medications or modalities without the guidance of trained medical personnel. In particular I cannot stress enough the importance of utilizing pain medications with great respect and with the guidance of medical professionals.

Everyone responds differently to different types of medications and it is important to understand this, as well as to know the potential side effects and complications associated with taking them. Even over-the-counter medications and supplements can cause severe damage to internal organs if not taken as advised. If you are unfamiliar with or are a first-time user of a new medication or supplement, always consult with your physician and pharmacist, and conduct your own research to understand how the medication might affect you.

A good patient must also understand that not every recommendation for pain management or physical therapy will work for them. You will have to become an educated consumer with respect to your health and try out different treatment options to help you manage your symptoms both pre-op and post-op. That includes both medication and physical therapy as well as alternative modalities. It may take weeks, months or even years to find the right combination of therapy that works for you. I encourage you to be proactive, ask lots of questions and, if needed, get a second opinion.

Medications

Prescription and OTC Pain Medications

I cannot begin to tell you how many medications and supplements I've tried to help ease the discomfort and pain of surgery both pre-op and post-op, including over fifty natural, homeopathic and over-the-counter products and natural nutritional supplements. In my efforts to avoid taking prescription pain medication I've experimented with just about every over-the-counter product you can imagine.

Unfortunately, I have found that prescription pain medication works the best for reducing discomfort and pain. Most of the OTC products and supplements did not work for me, or if they did, only slightly. I'm sure many of the products helped with my overall health, but they did nothing to combat severe pain.

It's also unfortunate that pharmaceutical companies have not yet developed pain medications which do not have serious side effects, including addiction. Scientists are currently working on developing newer drugs that do not have such side effects.

For my part, I have found that utilizing a combination of low-dose pregabalin, acetaminophen and ibuprofen works for me. I use medications sparingly and only when needed for what I consider permanent structural defects. This includes both acute and chronic pain from stenosis, arthritis, neuropathy and muscles spasms.

Early on in my treatment journey I was prescribed various medications. For example, I mentioned earlier that in 2012 my primary care doctor prescribed gabapentin for relief of my neuropathic pain before I could meet with an orthopedic surgeon for a follow-up diagnosis. This did the trick for the short time I was on it, helping me sleep and getting me through the next stage of the process leading up to ACDF surgery.

Following surgery, my physician recommended using pregabalin for pain-related symptoms from neuropathy. As always, I did my usual research on the medication before taking it. Pregabalin, brand name Lyrica, is classified as a miscellaneous analgesic and anticonvulsant under the Controlled Substances Act (CSA). According to Lyrica's website "Lyrica is indicated to treat fibromyalgia, diabetic nerve pain, spinal cord injury nerve pain and pain after shingles."[10]

Lyrica has many other off-label uses as well, including treating panic disorders, migraine prophylaxis, social phobia, mania, bipolar disorder, and alcohol withdrawal. Lyrica is also currently being studied as an add-on treatment for people who suffer from fibromyalgia, anxiety and depression. For me, Lyrica was a miracle and helped me manage most of my neuropathy and ACDF-related pain. (Later in this book I talk about maintaining your privacy regarding your treatment; as you can see from the list of uses for Lyrica, it would be easy for someone you're sharing your personal medical information with to misinterpret or second-guess your use of the drug for neuropathic peripheral nerve pain.)

Physicians and patients have to be careful how medications are prescribed and for what conditions, because health insurance companies have specific guidelines for using medications and may not cover "off label" use—in which case a patient would have to pay

---

[10] "For Some Patients, Lyrica Significantly Relieves Fibromyalgia Pain*." Lyrica, 2018, www.lyrica.com/?source=google&HBX_PK=s_lyrica&o=44962818%7C221361397%7C0&skwid=43700023461170844

out of pocket. I chose to try as many different alternatives as I could to avoid the use of opioid medications due to their side effects (including constipation—known as OIC—tolerance and the high risk of addiction). If you choose to use prescription opioids or OTC medication you will have to find out which products work best for you, but do so safely. Always be honest with and consult with your physician or pharmacist when taking any medication; your life may depend on it. Many medications have contraindications that you must pay close attention to. If you find yourself building a tolerance or becoming addicted to your pain medication, do not be embarrassed to ask for help right away. Any medical professional will be happy that you did.

Several physicians pointed out to me that more isn't always better with respect to the amount of medication a person takes. Only the smallest amount of medication necessary to relieve the symptoms of pain should be taken; this is the ultimate goal. Patients also have to worry about stressing their liver and kidneys. Any medication at high doses is toxic to the body; this includes OTC medication and supplements. Always know what type of medication you are taking, its possible side effects and its potential to interact with other drugs and supplements. Serious complications can occur, and risk of death is a real factor if medication is not taken as prescribed or is mixed with alcohol and/or other drugs, both prescription and illegal.

Opioids

I mentioned earlier that after my accident in 2006 I was prescribed two different opiates: Demerol and Vicodin (hydrocodone). This was to treat my pain immediately following the accident and surgery. Although they did their job at the time, I was very aware of the dangers of relying on them too much. Medications such as Demerol were only administered directly by the tending APRN under the surgeon's orders. I had been on hydrocodone for about eight weeks total, which included a three-week taper-off period so as not to experience PAWS (post-acute withdrawal syndrome). My physician told me, "I don't want you on this any longer than two months tops." I was similarly cautious when it came to managing my ACDF-related pain.

When seeking ways to manage pain it's probably best not to take the easy way out. I've witnessed both personally and professionally the outcomes for people who have sought pain relief and ended up abusing narcotic pain medications.

There are obviously pros and cons to taking opioid-based pain medications. The benefit, short term, is that they work almost immediately to eliminate most sensations of pain. So, as prescribed and for short periods of time, these medications have their place in the treatment of acute and severe chronic pain. The potential downside of taking opioid-based pain medications long-term is that they are highly addictive and also become less effective over time. This is a medical phenomenon called opioid-induced hyperalgesia (OIH). The body becomes overly sensitive to pain signals after using opioids for any length of time, and this decreases the medication's effectiveness, with patients needing to increase their dosage to get pain relief. Patients can quickly build up a tolerance and dependency, increasing the chances of addiction and other complications.

As an informed patient it is of the utmost importance to understand that anyone, regardless of their level of education or socioeconomic status, can become addicted to opioid-based pain medication. Addiction has affected many prominent and famous people. Stories of overdose and addiction flood the news daily, proving that no one is immune from this growing epidemic.

I have always had a great fear of and respect for pain medication. I think you should too. The descent to abuse and addiction can happen more easily and quickly than we think, even unknowingly. You must understand, respect and weigh the benefits versus the risks of taking opioid pain medications both short-term and long-term. If you take them, do so intelligently and only under the guidance of a medical professional.

It has been my experience that if a person must use pain medication it should be taken in the lowest dose possible for pain management, and for the shortest period of time. (Again, consult with your physician.) Sometimes pain medications are necessary and serve a much-needed purpose. With intelligent use and proper respect, using them doesn't have to be a life-altering event, and they can even be safely used long-term if needed, under a physician's care.

This is yet another reason why an open and honest relationship with your physician is paramount for your health.

Medical Marijuana and Other Medications

I am a huge proponent of the legalization and ethical use of medicinal marijuana for the treatment of pain as well as for other qualifying ailments. I have seen firsthand the benefits of its use on patients with chronic and severe injuries, including patients with incurable seizures, cancer and those who are overcoming post-traumatic stress disorder. Currently the legalization of marijuana and its beneficial and natural substances, such as cannabidiol (CBD) and tetrahydrocannabinol (THC) among many others, is on the rise throughout the United States. We must rid our society of the negative stigma of marijuana and other alternative and natural, plant-based healing substances. This will help us reduce or eliminate our dependency on dangerous pharmaceutical drugs like opioids.

(That said, I do not personally condone the use of recreational use of marijuana or any substance for "getting high" and numbing the pain of life's everyday obstacles and stressors. I believe a balanced

7: Pain Management Modalities

and holistic approach to its medicinal use is paramount.)

I am also a proponent of the ethical use and study of other natural and pharmacological medications to treat pain, such as ketamine, psilocybin, and other psychoactive chemicals. Physicians and scientists studying substances for medicinal use, including the management of pain must have a broad spectrum of available sources to select from to study. Limiting any substance, man-made or natural, that might safely help patients in pain is unethical. Currently, ketamine is being used to treat severe nerve pain, including neuropathy as well as other debilitating disorders. As our society and medical industry progresses towards a more holistic approach to alternative medicines, newer treatments and medications will become standard protocol in the treatment of pain, including ACDF-related pain and neuropathy.

Non-Medication Treatments

Myofascial Release Therapy

The fascia is a system of connective tissue mostly made of collagen which encases muscles and organs and helps support and maintain muscle grouping and separation. The fascia can also become a source of pain, which is generated by the nerves connected to the tissue, as well as by a tightening and rigidity of the tissue itself. This is called "myofascial pain."

This is a simple explanation of a much larger and more complex system which encases the muscular systems and groupings. I believe post-op myofascial pain is one component of the body's multi-faceted response to ACDF surgery. Myofascial release therapy is an effective, targeted method of manual massage and physical therapy, and it is one modality that can be used to help treat post-op related ACDF pain.

I have found that the post-op myofascial and muscle-related

trigger point pain and spasms I was experiencing from the "physiological relearning phase," were the most difficult to overcome. ("Physiological relearning phase" is a term I use to describe how cells and surrounding tissue that are disrupted during surgery adjust to their "new normal" after surgery.) I described my pain as a dull, annoying, pulling sensation on the back of the neck and radiating into the shoulders. When I was doing online research to find a solution to help manage my pain, I learned that many other patients who had undergone ACDF surgery experienced this same phenomenon.

Over time a numbness and tingling sensation began to settle in and radiated into my right shoulder and scapula blade area. I believe the neck muscles became fatigued from this relearning phase, and that this caused these symptoms. This type of myofascial pain and sensation continues to this day, although to a much lesser extent and at a far more manageable level. Some of this pain may be attributable to other cervical disc defects.

Nerve Ablation and Nerve Blocks

Nerve ablation and nerve blocks are methods used to destroy or deaden the nerve(s) responsible for sending pain signals to the brain, theoretically reducing or removing that pain. Nerve ablation is also known as radiofrequency ablation (RFA), cryoablation, neurotomy, or rhizotomy.

Radiofrequency ablation is accomplished using a special instrument to introduce high-frequency radio waves and create an electrical current. This current heats up the nerve, ablating it and interrupting pain signal output.[11] The cryoablation method utilizes a

---

[11] Leggett, Laura E, et al. "Radiofrequency ablation for chronic low back pain: A systematic review of randomized controlled trials." Pain Research &

similar specialized instrument to introduce cold, which freezes and ablates the nerve, reducing pain.[12] Although different ablation procedures utilize various methods and procedures to accomplish the ablation, the result is essentially the same.

With all this said, after doing my research I opted not to undergo the procedure. The patient reviews I read generally stated that the procedure was only a temporary solution, that it was risky, and that it did not have a great percentage of success. This was, of course, my own research and experience, and I encourage you to consult with your physician and research for yourself to see if you think the procedure is worth pursuing.

I *have* undergone nerve block injections with mixed results. These use a combination of anesthetic medication (usually lidocaine), steroids, epinephrine and pain medication to numb or reduce inflammation of the medial branch sensory nerves[13] in an effort to decrease sensory input and decrease pain. Personally, nerve block injections weren't as effective as I thought they would be for my ACDF-related pain. I also felt the risks outweighed the mild, if any, benefits I felt.

Physical Therapy and the McKenzie Method of Mechanical Diagnosis and Therapy

In my experience, physical therapy is not typically prescribed as part of the recovery process post-op ACDF. Unless a patient requests

---

Management: The Journal of the Canadian Pain Society, Pulsus Group Inc, 2014, www.ncbi.nlm.nih.gov/pmc/articles/PMC4197759/

[12] Lee, Thomas C. "MRI-Guided Cryoablation to Alleviate Pain in Head, Neck and Spine - Full Text View." Full Text View - ClinicalTrials.gov, 11 Feb. 2013, https://clinicaltrials.gov/ct2/show/NCT01788410

[13] Eckel, T S, and W S Bartynski. "Epidural steroid injections and selective nerve root blocks." Techniques in Vascular and Interventional Radiology., U.S. National Library of Medicine, Mar. 2009, http://www.ncbi.nlm.nih.gov/pubmed/19769903.

such therapy or the physician prescribes it, it does not seem to be considered a medically necessary treatment protocol for recovery. At least in my own case, no one told me that physical therapy might be highly beneficial to consider after surgery. I suggest that you look into it with your physician and see if there are elements of physical therapy that may help you.

For my part, one of the most effective ways I found to help manage my pain was "The McKenzie Method of Mechanical Diagnosis and Therapy"—also known as MDT. I discovered MDT while researching videos of physical therapy on YouTube. I came across a video of MDT discussing how it was helping patients who had severe scoliosis (curvature of the spine). The video showed children working with Dr. Robin McKenzie, a New Zealand-based physiotherapist who in the 1950s developed the MDT system.[14] After working with patients (mostly children) for several months he cured most of their conditions using only the physical therapy he'd developed, which strengthened and aligned the spine without the use of medication.

MDT therapy begins with an initial patient assessment, then goes on to classify the mechanical issues involved in the problem. The patient is also educated on avoiding future problems through an understanding of proper body function and posture. The major difference between MDT physical therapy and traditional physical therapy lies in how the joint is viewed as a mechanical, structural source of the problem. Traditional physical therapy utilizes stretching and strengthening of the limbs or muscles by various methods to bring them back to a normal range of mobility. MDT focuses on stretching and flexing the joint in a specific way to gain full flexion and mobility, as well as on strengthening the muscles supporting the joint. The

---

[14] "What Is the McKenzie Method?" The McKenzie Institute International®, www.mckenzieinstitute.org/patients/what-is-the-mckenzie-method/

focus on gaining full mechanical mobility and flexion of the joint is a key part of the process in eliminating radiating pain with respect to ACDF radiculopathy.

After seeing the video about MDT I began to conduct more research as to how it might relate to ACDF surgery and cervical issues. Once I decided that it could help, I researched diploma MDT therapists in my area and found a caregiver who was both a physical therapist and a certified McKenzie Mechanical Diagnostic therapist: Dr. Jonathan Dolutan. (There are different levels of MDT certification; an MDT diploma certification is the highest level of MDT training.)

One forty-five-minute session and a few home-stretching exercises later was all it took to mostly eliminate my constant radiating shoulder pain. During and immediately after my visit I was dumbfounded and told Dr. Dolutan I had gained additional range of motion and could no longer feel the radiating pain in my shoulder and neck. He laughed and told me that patients called him "the miracle man." He then further explained that our heads weigh approximately eleven pounds and rest in a forward position over the shoulders, which causes muscle fatigue and spasms. Add in technology—the way we talk on our phones and sit in front of our computers—and my recent ACDF surgery and pain made a lot more sense. Improper body posture leads to poor body alignment and causes a never-ending cycle of fatigue and pain.

He also told me that my cervical joints were stiff and had lost mobility. This was adding to the pain. The stretching and exercises I performed took that stress off the cervical nerves and joints; this helped decrease the pain and muscle fatigue. MDT, after only a few days, decreased my pain by 90 percent. I was amazed.

There is some discomfort when the movements are first started, and this is expected. As you perform the exercises and the cervical joints are stretched in an inverse position from their normal state, the joints are "relearning" their full range of mechanical motion, as well as relieving pressure on the nerves. We rarely stretch our joints to their full range of motion, so it is understandable that they will become stiff with a loss of range of motion.

I used acetaminophen and ibuprofen to help alleviate the discomfort I experienced the first few days after performing the physical therapy. After the third day the discomfort subsided.

If you have been diagnosed with cervical issues, such as protruding discs, stenosis, radiculopathy or degenerative arthritis-type issues and are considering surgery, also consider The McKenzie Method of Mechanical Diagnosis and Therapy, or physical therapy. It's my belief that minor issues with the cervical spine might be addressed and corrected with MDT—and without the intervention of surgery. A full evaluation by an MDT trained physical therapist will determine this. Even though I would not have personally benefited from MDT at the time of my diagnosis, I would highly recommend researching various physical therapy options that may benefit you. Despite being a primary candidate for surgery, I wish I'd known ahead of time about all the different treatments available to lessen my suffering.

In short, I am now a firm believer in physical therapy (MDT and other types) after ACDF surgery, and I feel this should be a mandatory part of the recovery process.

Cognitive Behavioral Therapy

In 2011 Luis Fernando Buenaver, Ph.D., an assistant professor of psychiatry and behavioral sciences at Johns Hopkins University School of Medicine published a study in *The Journal of Pain* entitled: "Evidence for indirect effects of pain catastrophizing on clinical pain among myofascial temporomandibular disorder participants: the mediating role of sleep disturbance."[15] Buenaver states in this paper, "If cognitive behavioral therapy can help people change the way they think about their pain, they might end that vicious cycle and feel better without sleeping pills or pain medicine." It has been my experience that constantly thinking about your pain will only make your pain worse. I found that keeping busy and engaging in activities that distracted me from ACDF-related pain were valuable coping methods that helped me manage my pain. Buenaver's paper can serve as a reminder that a skilled therapist may also play a role in pain management and recovery from ACDF surgery.

Lifestyle, Exercise and Diet

A healthy lifestyle, which includes nourishing foods and exercise, can definitely help to relieve pain. The importance of exercise and keeping the body moving cannot be underestimated. For me, exercise in any form, including physical therapy, yoga and massage, is the number one treatment of pain. It has both physical and psychological benefits.

I discovered that yoga had the biggest impact on my life with respect to relieving pain and overall psychological well-being. If you haven't discovered yoga, I suggest you look into it. Yoga strengthens and stretches all parts of the body as well as develops a sense of well-being. There are many different forms of yoga that anyone can do, even if you have severe health issues.

I also eat a healthy diet, take natural supplements, and try to limit caustic substances that increase inflammation, which include sugar,

---

[15] L. Buenaver, P. Quartana, M. Simango, E. Grace, R. Edwards, J. Haythornthwaite, M. Smith (2011). "Evidence for indirect effects of pain catastrophizing on clinical pain among myofascial temporomandibular disorder participants: the mediating role of sleep disturbance. The Journal of Pain, Vol. 12, Issue 4, P77, http://www.jpain.org/article/S1526-5900(11)00360-9/fulltext

alcohol, and processed junk food. I also eat foods that have analgesic properties, such as turmeric, ginger, pepper, and green leafy vegetables, as well as other fruits high in antioxidants, such as blueberries.

As noted above, I use medications sparingly and only when needed. For me this overall approach has worked best. I cannot stress the importance of exercise, stretching, and physical therapy and how positively it has impacted my overall constitution and well-being.

As with all the treatments discussed in this book, discuss yoga and other aspects of exercise and diet with your practitioner first. It is possible to injure yourself even with something as gentle as yoga, so is best to work with a highly trained yoga instructor initially to learn proper form and ensure you don't overdo your stretching.

Cold/hot Showers

The combination of hot and cold via hot showers or ice packs also helps to alleviate pain and reduce inflammation. Taking a hot shower is one of the first things I do to begin my day, and this helps loosen stiff and sometimes spasming muscles. The application of hot and cold to treat injuries is probably the oldest and simplest known medical treatment available, and sometimes the most effective.

Acupressure Mat

Another tool I use to help combat pain is an acupressure mat. This is a soft, flexible mat used to mimic the effects of acupuncture. When you lie on it, hundreds of pointed ends put pressure on the skin, stimulating increased blood flow and the release of natural hormones known as endorphins, which help alleviate pain. If you have sensitive skin or a low tolerance to pain, this may take some getting used to, but I have found it can work wonders. It is recommended that a beginner use the acupressure mat for only a few minutes at first, and then gradually increase the time as you get used to the new sensation.

7: Pain Management Modalities

TENS Units

There are a host of other devices and newer technologies that I have experimented with, including the use of a TENS (Transcutaneous Electrical Nerve Stimulation) unit. This is a small, pain-relieving electrical device which you can now purchase over-the-counter without a doctor's prescription. The TENS unit interrupts pain signals by sending small electrical impulses via electrodes to muscles that are spasming or in pain.

Cold Laser Therapy

I have also tried sessions of Cold Laser Therapy, also known as Low Level Laser Therapy (LLLT). This treatment is usually administered by a physical therapist. LLLT is a treatment modality that uses specific wavelengths of light that penetrate and interact with skin and muscle tissue and is thought to help alleviate pain by increasing blood flow to affected areas.[16]

Conclusion

As you can see, if your pain is severe and you are not getting relief from traditional treatment modalities or want to stay away from opioid-based medications, there are many other avenues for you to explore. I have touched on several in this chapter, but there are no doubt many other options available, and there will be more in the future. In addition to doing your own research, speak with your physician or pain management specialist about alternative treatments. Part of being an informed patient is familiarizing yourself with various safe and effective treatment options to put you in the best place to alleviate pain and live a happy and healthy life.

---

[16] Schnee A. Cold Laser Therapy Pain Management Treatment. Spine-health. 2009. Available at: https://www.spine-health.com/treatment/pain-management/cold-laser-therapy-pain-management-treatment. Accessed May 27, 2018.

Chapter 8

Health Insurance

Health Insurance Companies

It is estimated that the top six health insurance companies made approximately six billion dollars in profit in 2016 through 2017, up about 29 percent from the previous year.[17] Profits for insurance companies grew rapidly after the passage of the Patient Protection and Affordable Care Act of 2010, also known as the ACA and Obamacare.

Let me be clear on my position here: health insurance companies are big businesses designed to make one thing—money. The details of how they operate are complex and go well beyond the scope of this book. So the health insurance information discussed in this chapter relates specifically to my interactions with my health insurance provider with respect to undergoing ACDF surgery. One of the main points in my sharing some of these details is to alert you to some of the issues you will want to be aware of as you navigate your own journey. Ultimately every policy—and every individual—is different, so I recommend very strongly that you educate yourself on the ins and outs of your own health insurance coverage and policy.

---

[17] Coombs, Bertha. "As Obamacare twists in political winds, top insurers made $6 billion (not that there is anything wrong with that)." CNBC, CNBC, 6 Aug. 2017, www.cnbc.com/2017/08/05/top-health-insurers-profit-surge-29-percent-to-6-billion-dollars.html

Keep this question in mind: does your profit-driven health insurance company have your best interests in mind when providing you with health care services and processing your claims? I'll let you answer that.

Read Your Policy

Health care companies provide you with insurance against medical claims for sickness, injury, and general health check-ups, among other things. You or your employer usually pay a premium each month for health coverage under your health insurance policy.

Generally speaking, most people do not fully read or understand their health insurance policy. But the devil is in the details. As challenging or irritating as it may be for you to get clear on what's covered and what's not before seeking health care, it is vital for you to do so.

To offset their own costs, health insurance companies implement "cost sharing" in the form of co-pays, coinsurance and deductibles—essentially what you will pay on top of your monthly premium if you seek medical care. These kinds of cost sharing make things more expensive and complicated for patients to understand. And submitting claims and getting approval can be daunting.

Unfortunately, we need health insurance for general medical expenses and catastrophic events like surgery and medical care after an accident. As I'm sure you know, healthcare can be incredibly expensive. You and your family will need to plan for the burden of these expenses ahead of time—if you can. During an emergency surgical procedure for injury you may not have a choice but to proceed with whatever physicians recommend, regardless of whether you have the funds to pay for it.

There are things you can do right now concerning financial preparations to help you and your family avoid the stress associated with any pending surgery. First, take the time to fully read and understand your health insurance policy. If you need help with understanding and navigating the medical terminology and language within the policy, call the insurance company's help line or ask a family member or friend to see if they can go over it with you. If you have an insurance agent you can call them as well. If you have time and your surgery can be planned for, save extra money for all the associated costs you will have to bear on top of paying your monthly premium. This will make the process go more smoothly and remove some of the stress involved.

Pre-authorization

There are other health insurance issues to consider as well. These include understanding and ensuring proper authorization of pre-operative and post-operative medical services by your insurance company. Make certain that your policy covers every visit to your physician and each medical procedure you undergo. Many insurance companies require getting "pre-authorization" before you seek medical services or specialist appointments. And it does happen at times that they will not cover certain types of care. This is especially true when it comes to alternative treatments like acupuncture, but it can happen even with standard medical procedures. Many patients are in shock when they are denied services or claims by their health insurance company or are billed an exorbitant amount after receiving care. Again, it is important for you to read and fully understand your policy to make sure you do everything you need to do *before* you obtain the necessary services.

Many insurance companies use privately outsourced or third-party companies to approve medical procedures and claims. At the time of my ACDF surgery, my health insurance carrier utilized a third-party company known as National Imaging Associates, Inc., (NIA) to approve medical procedures and ensure they were medically necessary and fell within the guidelines set by the insurance company. I learned this the hard way after a medical procedure I was seeking was denied by NIA on behalf of my insurance company. I had been scheduled for a cervical ESI (epidural steroid injection) only to learn that my procedure was canceled the day it was supposed to take place.

Advocate for Yourself

Given all this, it is important for you to become your own advocate. Voice your concerns with respect to your rights within your insurance policy coverage and guidelines. If a procedure is denied, for example, you have the right to ask why and to request reconsideration. You can file a grievance with your physician, or take it up with your insurance company or any third-party acting on its behalf.

Your physician has the right to file what is known as a "peer review" with your insurance company or the third-party company. This is usually a documented medical report for reconsideration of services after a claim has been denied. Your physician will generate a detailed medical report for the insurance company or third-party entity to justify why the procedure is medically necessary for the patient.

So don't give up if a medical procedure or surgery is denied. Be persistent, make your voice heard and ask the right questions. After all, you are paying a high price for medical coverage, and there is a certain ethical responsibility that the insurance company has to you, their customer. All of this, too, is part of being an informed patient. Educating yourself on these issues can have an immediate and long-lasting impact not only on your physical well-being, but your financial well-being too.

Chapter 9

Medical Privacy

Your medical information is yours. Sometimes divulging too much of it can be detrimental to both your personal and professional life. I'm not talking here about the security of your personal and medical information, which has certain federal protections under the Health Insurance Portability and Accountability Act of 1996 (HIPPA). Rather in this chapter I want to briefly address how your personal medical information can be viewed with negative bias by family, friends, colleagues, employers and others.

Unfortunately, there is often a stigma attached to illness and injury, as well as to the use of medication. I know this not only from my personal experience, but also because it is a subject of research in medical journals. Many people view sickness as a weakness. Humans may in fact be biologically and psychologically wired to avoid those who are sick or ill. This bias may include individuals who are injured or recovering from surgery and who simply appear ill. For example, a study in the journal *Proceedings of the National Academy of Science* suggests that in the course of their evolutionary development, humans learned to detect subtle cues indicating someone might be ill—so that they could avoid those individuals in favor of their own biological fitness.[18]

Many prescription medications have a stigma associated with them. This is certainly true of opioids and medications used to treat mental health issues. One of the more subtle uses of language that reinforces this stigma is when we call prescription medications "drugs." The so-called "war on drugs" in the U.S. began in the 1970s, and since then public awareness about the abuse of illicit and prescription medications has grown. One side effect of this is that the word "drugs"—even when used to refer to prescription medications taken correctly—is often associated with something illicit. That is, if you're on "drugs" there's something wrong with you. Of course, not everyone consciously believes this, but this subtle, subconscious association exists.

What can we take away from these thoughts? Although at times we feel the need to express what we are experiencing, especially after something as significant as major surgery, we should also be aware that the information we provide to others through general conversation may not be received in the way we'd like it to be. Not everyone will be interested or sympathetic, and whatever we share can color the view that a person holds of us. I am not saying that everyone will behave this way—there are many compassionate individuals in the world. I am only suggesting that you consider carefully who you share your personal health information with.

Here is a small personal example. I was discussing my ACDF surgery with a friend of mine, whom I'll call Tom. He had undergone ACDF surgery about two years after me. I asked Tom if he'd had any ongoing pain issues post-op. He told me that he'd gone through the typical recovery phase pain and was a little sore, but had only needed

---

[18] Regenbogen, C., Axelsson, J., Lasselin, J., Porada, D., Sundelin, T., Peter, M., Lekander, M., Lundström, J. and Olsson, M., Behavioral and neural correlates to multisensory detection of sick humans, May 22, 2017.
https://www.pnas.org/content/114/24/6400

prescription medication for a few days out of surgery. After that he used acetaminophen to manage his post-op pain.

Tom had had a one-level ACDF procedure; he'd had no other complications or relevant medical history. My own condition was a bit more complex. When he asked about my experience, I explained that I'd had a bit more pain post-op from the surgery than him, and that I was also trying to manage the pain from another cervical level injury, as well as femoral nerve damage pain from the broken hip I sustained during my accident. As we talked, I could tell that Tom was being negative and judgmental towards me.

Afterwards I wished I had kept my information to myself. I had assumed he would be more open-minded and accepting of what I was going through, but I was wrong. Not only had he not seemed to consider the differences in our underlying conditions, but he also felt the need to lecture me. The incident made me wonder what my co-workers would think. Would they see me as a liability—or even worse, engage in malicious gossip—if they knew about my ongoing medical condition?

Ultimately this encounter taught me a lesson: some people, even friends, can be extremely judgmental and opinionated when it comes to another person's health issues. As a consequence, I no longer openly share my personal health information, even with close friends.

The bottom line is that your health condition can be seen as a potential liability or weakness. If you value your privacy and want to limit collateral damage from gossip and judgement by others, you might want to keep your private medical information private. At the very least, consider deeply who you choose to share this aspect of your life with.

Chapter 10

Healthy Living

I'm sure you've heard the phrase, "body, mind, and spirit." Together the words refer to the areas in one's life that we can all pay more attention to in order to live a healthy and fulfilling life. Part of living a healthy lifestyle is having a positive attitude and realizing that life is a gift from God that should not be wasted. Although this book is primarily about the nuts and bolts of ACDF surgery, I wanted to write this brief chapter to make it clear that I believe a positive attitude and healthy lifestyle will go a long way to helping you on your ACDF journey.

Many ancient people lived simply and did not possess the same ills that we have in modern times. Ancient people were more in tune with their being, constitution and health. Today we have many modern "sicknesses" that often result from poor posture—often due to the overuse of technology—and living a sedentary lifestyle. Also common is the the abuse of legal and recreational drugs, including alcohol. (A recent paper in the *Journal of the National Comprehensive Cancer Network* detailing a correlation between alcohol consumption and cancer is alarming.[19])

---

[19] Sanford, Nina N., David J. Sher, Xiaohan Xu, Chul Ahn, Anthony V. D'Amico, Ayal A. Aizer, and Brandon A. Mahal. "Alcohol Use Among Patients With Cancer and Survivors in the United States, 2000–2017", *Journal of the National Comprehensive Cancer Network J Natl Compr Canc Netw.* 18, 1: 69-79.

Ancient people also held deep spiritual beliefs, which I believe helped them maintain a healthy attitude and lifestyle. They knew that individual acts of selfishness could potentially put the entire tribe at risk.

In the modern world it seems to be more difficult to find that sense of community and individual connectedness. I feel strongly about living a healthy lifestyle and believe that if you take care of your body, the mind and spirit will prosper. All bodily systems are connected and need to be kept in concert to keep everything in balance. As with a mechanical device like a car, if one part fails it usually affects the entire system.

The Greek physician Hippocrates has been credited with the saying, "Let thy food be thy medicine, and let thy medicine be thy food." This is a good axiom to consider regarding your health. What you eat and put into your body is extremely important. Food is the fuel that keeps your body healthy, and the types of foods you eat directly impact your health. Eating a natural, healthy, balanced diet should be your first priority. It will help you feel better in all areas of your life, and you will not burden your body with the challenges of dealing with and eliminating the toxins in modern processed foods. This will help your body heal faster and boost your psychological well-being; this in turn will have a positive impact on your relationships with others. Soon after my surgery I began to examine my diet closely and did my best to cut out unhealthy food and drink, especially sugar.

After you have addressed your dietary concerns, exercise should be your next consideration following recovery from surgery. A sedentary lifestyle leads to all sorts of medical problems and negatively affects your mindset and psychological well-being. Living a sedentary life after surgery can also lead to depression and anxiety; exercise and diet are the number-one remedies physicians consider when treating these disorders.

As you can see it is extremely important to take personal inventory of your current health and well-being and make changes accordingly. Eating healthy, exercising, and living a healthy lifestyle not only affect how you feel, but also positively impacts the relationships you have with others. It prepares your body, mind and spirit to respond to whatever challenges come your way.[20] Ultimately you have the power within yourself to make these changes in your life.

---

[20] As a side note, I write this during the COVID-19 events of 2020, a time during which being in the best possible state of health is crucial to assist the body to fight infections.

Chapter 11

Reflections on Being an Informed Patient

Intelligent preparation for ACDF surgery impacts the entire process from beginning to end. It can help things go well, and if unexpected events occur, proper planning can put you in a better position to understand and mitigate any problems that arise. Becoming an informed patient enhances one's chances for a speedy recovery and can also, I believe, alleviate some of the psychological stress we feel when facing the unknown.

All that said, I understand that some people may not want to know all the details of their surgery. That's okay, too, though if you're feeling uncertainty or fear around the idea of surgery—very normal feelings for anyone—I invite you to explore whether the idea of becoming better informed might actually address that fear.

Currently, post-op seven years, I continue to adhere to my own advice: living healthy, eating healthy and exercising. I have become aware of my body's needs, including sleep and water—two of the most overlooked requirements for health. I believe that all of these choices are helping the current state of my neck, maintaining the stability of the surgical site post-op and, I hope, helping me lessen the need for a possible future surgery of other affected cervical discs. Overall, I can state that my body is in a healthy and balanced position to overcome most health obstacles.

Everyone processes life's obstacles differently and in their own way. The most important lesson I've learned is to be my own advocate. No one is better at taking care of me than me. I also learned that keeping a positive attitude is an extremely important aspect of dealing with stress and managing pain.

In a sense, those who have had ACDF surgery will be ACDF "patients for life." This might mean for some that they have some minor restriction in movement, some residual pain or scarring, or simply the memory of the experience and its impact on their lives. Acknowledging this can relieve a lot of anxiety and stress. Keeping a positive attitude will help you manage your condition and pain.

Undergoing ACDF surgery is a life-altering event. How you go about the process is very important. If you are facing this prospect, I encourage you to learn as much as you can about the surgery and recovery process. Ultimately, you're responsible for making your own health decisions. I'm grateful for all the experiences and people I've met along the way and for those who helped me throughout my surgery and recovery. In the end the experience made me more appreciative of my life. Whatever decisions you make, remember to be positive, live a healthy lifestyle, be nice to those around you—especially your family—and when you need help, ask for it!

Good luck on your own path to recovery.

Glossary

Acetaminophen

A pain-relieving analgesic medication also known as paracetamol or APAP; its common brand name is Tylenol.

ACDF

Anterior Cervical Discectomy and Fusion.

Acute

When used to refer to illness or pain, an abrupt and quick onset, versus a chronic condition.

Analgesic

A medicine, either natural or synthetic, that reduces the sensation of pain.

Anesthesia

A drug usually used during surgery to induce a deep state of sleep in which the patient is unaware of conscious perception and pain.

Anesthesiologist

Physicians/doctors who specialize in the field of anesthesiology.

Anesthesiology

The study and practice of methods to reduce or relieve pain during surgery. As discussed in this book it refers particularly to the "general" anesthesia used during the ACDF procedure, as opposed to "local" anesthesia of the type used, for example, during minor dental procedures.

Anterior

Referring to a location "before" or toward the front of something.

APRN

Advanced Practice Registered Nurse.

Arthritis

Joint disease.

Cervical

Of or relating to the neck or cervix.

Consultation

A meeting with a physician or surgeon to discuss current medical conditions and options relating to a patient's health.

CSA

Controlled Substances Act

Demerol

Brand name of the pain prescription drug meperidine hydrochloride.

Diagnosis

The process of determining which disease or condition explains a person's symptoms and signs. [Source: Wikipedia]

Diazepam

Medication of the benzodiazepine family used as a calming agent, muscle relaxant, and to aid in a range of other illnesses.

Discectomy

The surgical removal of herniated disc material.

Disc Degeneration

Also referred to as "degenerative disc disease," this occurs in the spine and is caused by a natural breakdown of intervertebral discs due to trauma, overuse, and disease.

Disc Protrusion

Also referred to as a "bulging disc" occurring within the spinal vertebrae. It is usually caused by trauma or degenerative conditions.

EMT

Emergency Medical Technician.

ER

Emergency Room, located in a hospital, an ER usually tends to patients in need of immediate medical attention.

ESI

Epidural Steroid Injection.

Fascia

Tissue that connects or encloses muscles and internal organs.

Fracture

Broken bone, medical condition in which there is a damage in the continuity of the bone. [Source: Wikipedia]

Fusion

The joining and fusing of two bones, spinal fusion, also called spondylodesis or spondylosyndesis, is a neurosurgical or orthopedic surgical technique that joins two or more vertebrae. [Source: Wikipedia]

Gabapentin

Prescription anticonvulsant medication used to treat nerve pain, seizures and other disorders.

GP

General practitioner, a physician practicing in general or family medicine.

Hydrocodone

A semi-synthetic opioid used to treat severe pain.

Ibuprofen

A nonsteroidal anti-inflammatory drug (NSAID) class pain medication.

Interbody device

Man-made prosthetic device usually made of different forms of metal and/or special plastics used in spinal fusions.

Intervertebral disc

A disc-shaped fibrocartilaginous joint (a joint connected by both fibrous and cartilaginous tissue) in between each individual spinal vertebra.

Intubation

Medical procedure usually performed by an anesthesiologist, nurse anesthetist or respiratory therapist during surgery utilizing an endotracheal tube (ET) through the mouth of the patient to keep the airway open and deliver oxygen during surgery.

MD

Medical doctor, physician.

Medication

Any man-made or natural substance used as a drug for medical treatment.

Modality

Relating to medical terminology, usually a therapeutic method.

MRI

Magnetic Resonance Imaging.

MRI machine
MRI (Magnetic Resonance Imaging) machines create detailed images utilized by physicians to help make medical diagnoses.

MTBI
Mild traumatic brain injury.

Myelopathy
An injury related to the nerves in the spinal cord.

Myofascial
Relating to the fasciae (connective tissue) of muscles.

Narcotic
In modern usage, an opioid-based drug (either natural or synthetic) used to relieve pain.

Neurologist
A physician specializing in neurology.

Neurology
A branch of medicine dealing with disorders of the nervous system. [Source: Wikipedia]

Neuropathic pain
Pain related to damage to nerves and the nervous system.

Nociceptive pain
Pain arising from the stimulation of nerve cells.

NPO
Nil Per Os in Latin or nothing by mouth.

NSAID
Nonsteroidal anti-inflammatory drugs used to reduce inflammation; common versions include Advil and Aleve and Aspirin.

OIC

Opioid Induced Constipation.

Opioid

A type of natural and/or synthetic drug derived or synthesized from the opium plant that is used primarily for pain relief.

Orthopedics/Orthopedic Surgery

The branch of surgery concerned with conditions involving the musculoskeletal system. [Source: Wikipedia]

OTC medication

"Over-the-counter" medicine or supplements that can be purchased at a pharmacy without a prescription.

PA

Physician's Assistant.

PACU

Post Anesthesia Care Unit.

Paralysis

Loss of muscle function of one or more muscles.

Pathophysiology

The disordered physiological processes associated with disease or injury. [Source: Wikipedia]

PCP

Primary Care Physician.

Pharmacist

A healthcare professional who practices in the medical field of pharmacy, which focuses on the safe and effective use of medication.

PMP

Pain Management Physician.

Post-operative or post-op
After surgery.

Pseudarthrosis/nonunion
A permanent failure of healing following a broken bone unless intervention (such as surgery) is performed. [Source: Wikipedia]

Psychosomatic disorder
A disease which involves both mind and body.

PT
Physical therapist or physical therapy.

Pulmonary aspiration
Inhalation of food, liquids, vomit or other substances into the lungs or airways.

Radiculopathy
Also commonly known as a "pinched nerve," radiculopathy is a mechanical compression or irritation of the nerves as they exit the intervertebral foramen. Radiculopathy usually causes pain, numbness and a tingling sensation in the affected area.

Radiologist
A medical doctor who specializes in using medical imaging techniques such as x-rays and magnetic resonance imaging to diagnose disease.

Referred Pain
Pain perceived at a location in the body other than where the pain actually originates. [Source: Wikipedia]

Shock
Psychological shock or acute stress reaction to any stressful event.

Spine
Vertebral column, also known as the backbone, part of the axial

skeleton. [Source: Wikipedia]

Stenosis (spinal)

Compression or narrowing of the channel through which the nerves run in the spine, often due to trauma or arthritis.

Surgeon

A physician who performs surgery. [Source: Wikipedia]

TBI

Traumatic brain injury.

Trauma

Can refer to acute physical injury or psychological distress.

Unconsciousness

The absence of conscious awareness, usually resulting in the inability to respond to environmental stimuli.

Vertebra

In the vertebrate spinal column, each vertebra is an irregular bone with a complex structure composed of bone and some hyaline cartilage, the proportions of which vary according to the segment of the backbone and the species of vertebrate. [Source: Wikipedia]

Vicodin

Brand name for a pain medication that is a mix of hydrocodone and paracetamol.

X-Ray, X-Ray machine

X-radiation, a form of electromagnetic radiation given off from an X-ray machine that can penetrate skin and other substances to varying depths, and which is used in medical diagnosis.

Index

#
3 Tesla magnet, 35

A
ablation procedures, 79
ACA (Affordable Care Act of 2010), 87
accident, 16, 23–28, 74, 88, 95
  history of the author's, 26
  six years after, 27
ACDF club, 18
ACDF fusion surgery
  accident that caused, 23–27
  aftermath of, 31, 54, 55, 56, 61, 78, 80, 99, 109
  basic concepts of, 19
  choice of surgeon for, 41–52
  diagnosis, 11, 16–18, 26–28, 29–39, 44, 73, 80–82, 104, 110
  explanation about, 15–21
  glossary about, 103–110
  health insurance and, 87–91
  and healthy living post-op, 97–99
  history of, 16
  hospital stay and, 54
  informed patient and, 101–102
  a life-altering event, 102
  managing pain and, 64–69
  and medical privacy, 93–95
  medications and, 72–77
  non-medication treatments and, 77–85
  preparation for, 50, 101
  quantity of, 16
  reaction to diagnosis of, 42
  realizing the need for, 42
  risks of, 19–20, 44, 46
  post-op and, 53–62
  pre-op (two weeks prior to), 50
  signs and symptoms, 27–28
  surgeon choice for, 43–45
  summary of treatment modalities, 85
  what to expect from, 16–17, 19, 21, 42
  Zagata, Dr. Mateusz, and, 11–12
ACDF-related pain, 65, 67, 73, 75, 77, 79, 83
acetaminophen, 27, 61, 72, 82, 95, 103
ACL, torn, 58
acupressure mat, 84–85
acupuncture, 65, 85, 89
addiction, 64, 72, 74, 75, 76
Advanced Practice Registered Nurse (APRN), 17, 75, 104
Advil, 27, 107
advocate for yourself, 20, 21, 90
alcohol, 49–50, 73–74, 84, 97
Aleve, 107
alleviate pain, 71–85

allograft, 48–50
alternative medicines, 77
amnesia, 52
amnesic syndrome, 52
analgesic, 26, 73, 84, 103
ancient people, lifestyle and beliefs of, 97–98
anesthesia, 51, 53, 54, 55, 56, 103, 108
anesthesiologist, 20, 51–52, 53, 54, 103, 106
anesthesiology, 103
anesthetic medication, 79
anterior, 104
anterior cervical discectomy and fusion (ACDF). See ACDF fusion surgery.
anti-anxiety medication, 61
anticonvulsant medication, 30, 61, 73, 105
anxiety, 52, 53, 61, 63, 73, 99, 102
APAP (acetaminophen), 103
appointments, trusted third party and, 68
APRN (Advanced Practice Registered Nurse), 17, 75, 104
arthritis, 27, 58, 72, 104, 110
articulations, 32, 36
aspirin, 107
autologous graft (autograft), 48
axial skeleton, 110

B
backbone, 110
before surgery consultation, 50
belief perseverance, 38

benzodiazepenes/benzodiazepine 52, 104
blood panel, full, 51
blood tests, 50, 51
board certified physician, 11, 45
body alignment, poor, 81
body moving, importance of, 83
body posture, improper, 81
bone, irregular, 110
brain injury, mild traumatic (MTBI), 24, 107
Buenaver, Luis Fernando, Ph.D., 83
bulging disc, 42, 105

C
C3 (cervical vertebrae 3), 24
C6–C7 level, 30, 42
calcification, 35
calming agent, 104
cannabidiol (CBD), 76
cartilage, 110
cartilaginous, 106
case history, 23–28
catastrophic events, 88
CBC (Complete Blood Count), 51
CBD (cannabidiol), 76
cervical
  brace, 59
  condition, ongoing, 28
  disc protrusion, 66
  ESI (epidural steroid injection), 90
  interbody device, 46
  issues, 30, 60, 81–82
  joints, 81–82

Index

lordosis, 33, 36–37
neuropathy, 66
radiculopathy, 29
spinal fusion surgery, 12
spine (neck), 16, 24, 32, 35, 38, 41, 48, 82
surgery, 16
vertebrae and discs, 26
choosing a surgeon, process of, 43
chronic condition, 103
chronic pain, 25, 67–68, 72, 75
side effects of, 68
co-pays, 88
co-sufferers, 68
coagulation study test, 51
codeine, 25
cognitive behavioral therapy, 83
coinsurance, 88
Cold Laser Therapy Pain Management Treatment, 85n
cold/hot showers, 84
Cole, Dr., 48
communicating with your family, 68
complacency, 20
Complete Blood Count (CBC), 51
complications
after surgery, 19, 37, 41, 44, 47–50, 54, 58, 62, 95
potential, 47
serious, 74
compression, 29, 30, 37, 49, 109, 110
concussion, symptoms of, 25
confirmation bias, 38

conscious awareness, absence of, 110
constipation, 74
consultation, 11, 16, 28, 41–52, 104
Controlled Substances Act (CSA), 73, 104
coping methods, 68, 83
cost sharing, 88
co-pays, 88
COVID-19 events of 2020, 99
craniovertebral junction (CVJ), 32, 35
cryoablation, 78, 79
CSA (Controlled Substances Act), 73, 104

D
dangers of opioids, 26, 64, 75
Davidson, Dr. Mark, 43, 45–47, 49–52
debilitating disorders, 77
deductibles, 88
degenerative disc disease, 33, 37, 104
degenerative disc pathology, 16
Demerol, 24, 57, 74, 75, 104
denial, 19
dependency on pharmaceutical drugs, 64, 77
depression, 63, 73, 99
diagnosis
initial, 29, 31, 33, 35, 37, 39
proper, 16–17, 38–39
diagnostic
imaging, 38
process and surgery, 39
radiology image report, 32, 35

testing, problems with, 38
diazepam, 51–52, 53–54, 104
diet, 99
dietary concerns, 98
dihydrocodeine, 25
disc degeneration, 27, 104
disc protrusion (bulging disc), 27, 32–33, 36, 42, 66, 105
discectomy, 12, 15–16, 32–33, 35–36, 38, 103–104
documentation, 21
Dolutan, Dr. Jonathan (physical therapist), 81
driving after surgery, 54
drugs
  abuse of, 97
  legal and recreational, 97
  newer, 72
  war on, 94
dysphasia, 55–56

E
eating healthy, 50, 99, 101
educate yourself, 12, 21, 87, 91
educated consumer, 71
electromagnetic radiation, 110
Emergency Medical Technician (EMT), 17, 105
emergency room, 23–24, 105
EMT (Emergency Medical Technician), 17, 105
endorphins, 85
endotracheal tube (ET), 51, 53, 106
epidural steroid injection (ESI), 67, 90, 105
epinephrine, 79

ESI (epidural steroid injection), 67, 90, 105
exercise, 61, 65, 83–84, 98–99, 101
  psychological benefits of, 83
exercises, 81

F
family doctor, 27, 67, 68
family
  communicating with, 68
  support from, 68
fascia/fasciae (connective tissue), 65, 77, 105, 107
fibrocartilaginous joint, 106
fibromyalgia, 73
financial preparations, 89
fissure, 33, 36
foci (points of interest), 35
food, 50, 53, 84, 98, 109
  as medicine, 98
  nourishing, 83
foraminal narrowing, 32, 33, 36, 37
fracture, 24, 58, 105
fusion (defined), 105

G
gabapentin, 30, 73, 105
general practitioner (GP), 20, 66, 67–68, 105
  advantages of choosing, 67–68
glossary of medical terminology, 17
glucose test, 51
going home, 60

Index

GP (general practitioner), 20, 66, 67–68, 105
grievance, file a, 90

H
hardware and implant options, 47
heads, weight of, 81
heal faster, 98
health, requirements for, 101
health care companies, 88
health check-ups, general, 88
health coverage, 88
health insurance, 19, 20, 21, 50, 60, 67, 73, 87–91, 93
  companies, 73, 87–88
  information, 87
  policy, 88–89
Health Insurance Portability and Accountability Act of 1996 (HIPPA), 93
health-related issues, 58
healthcare, incredible expense of, 60, 88
healthy attitude, 98
healthy lifestyle/living, 83, 97–99, 102
helmet, 23
herniated disc, 104
HIPPA (Health Insurance Portability and Accountability Act of 1996), 93
Hippocrates, 14, 98
holistic approach, 77
homeopathic, 72
hormones, 85
hospital, overnight stay at, 54
hyaline cartilage, 110
hydrocodone (generic Vicodin), 25, 30, 57–58, 74–75, 106, 110
hyperalgesia, 63, 75
hypersensitive, 63
hypertrophy, 32, 33, 36, 37

I
ibuprofen, 27, 61, 72, 82, 106
iliac crest, 48
image, informative, 35
imaging, 24, 27, 32, 35, 38, 90, 106–107, 109
imaging technology, newer, 27
implant, 46–48
individual connectedness, 98
inflammation, 30, 64, 79, 84, 107
information
  gathering, 41
  useful, 66
  we provide to others, 94
informed patient, 12–13, 16–18, 20–21, 24, 26, 28, 30–32, 34, 36, 38, 42, 44, 46, 48, 50, 52, 54, 56, 58, 60, 62, 64, 66, 68, 72, 74–76, 78, 80, 82, 84, 85, 88, 90–91, 94, 98, 101–102, 104, 106, 108, 110
initial diagnosis, 29, 31, 33, 35, 37, 39
initial incision, 58
injury/injuries, 11, 20, 23–24, 26–27, 30, 35–36, 50, 58, 64, 73, 88, 93, 95, 107–108, 110
  misdiagnosed, 26
  understanding your own, 26
insurance agent, 89
insurance claims, 21

getting approval for, 67, 88
submitting, 88
insurance premium, 88–89
intact (not damaged or impaired), 36
interbody device, 46–47, 106
internal organs, severe damage to, 71
intervention, 25, 66, 82, 109
intervertebral disc, 37, 106
intravertebral graft, 32
intubation, 51, 106

J
joint disease, 104
Journal of Pain, The, 83

K
ketamine, 77

L
lidocaine, 79
living healthy, 101
LLLT (Low Level Laser Therapy), 85
loved ones becoming victims, 69
Low Level Laser Therapy (LLLT), 85
Lyrica, 73
off label uses of, 73–74

M
magnetic resonance imaging (MRI), 21, 24, 30–36, 39, 41–42, 79, 106–107, 109
mainstream medicine, 64
malaise, general, 61

managing pain, 59–60, 63, 54, 65, 67, 69, 102
marijuana, 76–77
legalization of, 76
negative stigma of, 76
massage, 27–28, 62, 78, 83
manual, 78
neck, 18
therapist, 28
McKenzie Institute International®, 80
Mckenzie method (MDT), 80–82
McKenzie, Dr. Robin, 80
MDT (McKenzie Method of Mechanical Diagnosis and Therapy), 80–82
mechanical motion, full range of, 82
medical advice, 4, 17–18, 45
medical care after an accident, 88
medical diagnosis, 110
medical expenses, general, 88
medical history, 29, 39, 45, 48, 51, 95
medical imaging techniques, 109
medical information, 30, 45, 73, 93, 95
federal protections of, 93
personal, 73, 93
private, 95
medical language, 103–110
medical privacy, 93–95
medical problems, various, 98
medical procedure/surgery denied, 90

Index

medical terms/terminology, 17, 103–110
medical/medicinal marijuana, 76
medications
  addictive, 52, 75
  contraindications of, 74
  patient liaison and, 21
  prescription pain, 18, 24, 25–26, 52, 54, 56–57, 61, 64, 65, 71–76, 94, 95, 104, 105, 110
  safe and effective use of, 108
  stigma with using, 93
  stressing liver and kidneys, 74
  use of, 80, 93, 108
  using sparingly, 84
  for mental health, 94
medicine as food, 98
meditation, 65
Medtronic Inc. (company), 46–48
mental health, medications for, 94
meperidine/meperidine hydrochloride, 57, 104
miracle man, 81
misdiagnosed, 26
modalities of treatment, 19, 58, 65, 71–73, 75, 77, 78, 79, 81, 83, 85, 106
modalities, alternative, 72
morphine/morphine sulfate, 56
morphology, 32, 35
motor deficit, 42
movement, minor restriction in, 102

MRI (magnetic resonance imaging), 21, 24, 30–36, 39, 41–42, 79, 106–107, 109
MRI radiology report, 35–39
MTBI (mild traumatic brain injury), 24, 107
multilevel fusion, 42
multiplanar imaging, multisequence, 32, 35
muscle impairment, 29
muscle relaxant medication, 61, 104
muscles spasms, 72
muscles, atrophy of, 61
musculoskeletal system, 108
myelopathy, 29, 49, 107
myofascial
  defined, 107
  pain, 28, 77–78, 83
  release therapy, 77–78

N
narcotic, 75, 107
National Imaging Associates, Inc. (NIA), 90
natural healing force, 14
natural nutritional supplements, 72
neck brace, 59
neck pain, 16, 23–24, 26–27, 32, 35
  chronic, 16
negative outcomes, 53
nerve ablation, 78
nerve block injections, risks of, 79
nerve blocks, 78, 79

nerve impingement, 27, 30–31, 42
nerve pain
 diabetic, 73
 neuropathy caused, 30
 severe, 77
neural foramina, 32–33, 36
neurological impairment, 29
neurological symptoms, 47
neurologist/neurology, 107
neuropathic pain, 30, 64, 73, 107
neuropathy, 30, 49, 57, 64, 66, 72–73, 77, 107
 debilitating aspects of, 30
 pain-related symptoms from, 73
neurospine surgeons, 41
neurosurgeon or orthopedic surgeon?, 43, 105
neurotomy, 78
new normal, 65, 78
newer drugs, 72
nil per os (NPO), 53, 107
nociceptive, 63–64, 107
non-medication treatments, 77
nonsteroidal anti-inflammatory drug (NSAID), 27, 28, 106, 107
nonunion, 109
normal feelings, 101
nothing by mouth (NPO), 53, 107
NPO (nil per os), 53, 107
NSAID (nonsteroidal anti-inflammatory drug), 27, 28, 106, 107
numbness and tingling, 16, 29, 78, 109
nurse anesthetist, 106
nurses, 17, 20, 54, 104, 106
 being nice to, 57
nutrition, 65
nutritional supplements, 65, 72

O

Obamacare (ACA), 87
OIC (Opioid Induced Constipation), 74, 108
one-level ACDF procedure, 95
opiate/opiates, 57, 74
opioid crisis, 67
Opioid Induced Constipation (OIC), 108
opioid medications, 25, 26, 57, 75, 85, 107
 and addiction high risk, 74, 75
 avoid use of, 74
 benefits of, 26, 76
 dangers and risks of, 26, 75, 76
 pros and cons, 75
 tolerance of, 74
opioid-based analgesic pain medication. *See* opioid medications.
opioid-based drug, 107
opioid-induced hyperalgesia (OIH), 75
opioids, 25, 26, 57, 67, 74, 75, 76, 77, 85, 94, 106, 107, 108. *See also* opioid medications.
opium plant, 108
opium poppy, 25
options
 for alleviating pain, 65
 for choice of surgeons and surgery, 41–52

Index

consultation and, 104
long-term care, 19
for pain management, 71–85
for pain treatment, 64–65, 67, 71
physical therapy, 82
quality of life, 19
orthopedic spine surgeon, 30, 41–43, 44, 45, 59, 73
board-certified, 30, 44
consultation with, 41–52
follow-up diagnosis and, 73
professionalism and care, 62
specializes in, 30
orthopedics/orthopedic surgery, 108
OTC (over-the-counter) medications, 27, 61, 65, 72, 74, 108
OTC (over-the-counter) supplements, 71
outpatient ambulatory surgery, 60
over-the-counter (OTC) supplements, 71

P

PACU (post anesthesia care unit), 55, 108
pain, 11, 16–19, 23–30, 32, 35, 38, 42, 47, 51, 55–61, 63–69, 71–85, 94–95, 102–110
acute, 24, 25, 29, 55, 58, 63–64, 66, 72, 75, 103
acute and/or chronic, 25, 63–64, 72, 75
back, 11
basic concepts of, 64
becoming addicted to, 74
chronic, 25, 67–68, 72, 75
constant and increasing, 29
controlled by, 66
easing it between appointments, 30
escape from by suicide, 66
excruciating and unbearable, 66
informed patient and, 64
issues, ongoing, 94
managing between appointments, 30
and muscle spasms, 38
nature of, 63
neck, 11, 16, 23–24, 26–27, 32, 35
number one treatment of, 83
phenomena of, 63
physiology of, 64
recovery phase, 94
severe, 30, 58, 66, 72, 77, 106
symptomatic, 42
types of, 63, 66
unbearable, 28, 66
understanding and managing, 59, 63, 65, 67, 69
pain level, 66
7–8 out of 10, 66
pain management, 11, 56, 61, 64, 67, 69, 71–85, 109
chronic or post-operative, 67
healthy ways of, 66
modalities, 71, 73, 75, 77, 79, 81, 83, 85
physician (PMP), 65, 67, 109
safe, 64–65, 78, 80, 83

specialist, 67, 85
pain medication, 18, 24, 25–26, 27–28, 52, 54, 56–57, 61, 64, 65, 66, 71–76, 77, 79, 80, 84, 85, 94, 95, 103, 104, 105, 106, 108, 110
  becoming addicted to, 74
  fear of, 64
  relying too much on, 61
pain relief, 75, 108
pain scale method, standard medical, 66
pain scales, 66
pain threshold, personal, 56
pain-related symptoms from neuropathy, 73
pain-relief approaches, alternative and natural, 64
pain-relieving electrical device, 85
paracentral disc, 33, 36
paracetamol, 103, 110
paralysis, 19, 23, 29, 53, 108
patent (defined), 36
pathophysiology, 55, 63, 108
patient assessments, 27
patient liaison, 21
Patient Protection and Affordable Care Act of 2010, 87
patients for life, 102
PAWS (Post-Acute Withdrawal Syndrome), 75
PCP (phenylcyclohexylpiperidine), 25, 29–30, 65, 108

PCP (primary care physician), 25, 29–30, 67, 108
PEEK Prevail® system, 46–48
peer review, 90
peripheral nerve pain, 73
personal health information, sharing 94
personal interview, 51
pharmaceutical companies, 72
pharmacist, 71, 74, 108
pharmacy, 108
physical injury, acute, 110
physical therapist, 20, 81, 82, 85, 109
physical therapy, 65, 71–72, 78, 80–84, 109
  traditional, 80
physician choice, 66-67
physician, experienced, 27
physiological relearning phase, 78
physiotherapist, 80
pinched nerve, 109
planning, proper, 101
plant-based healing substances, 76
Plous, Scott, 38
PMP (Pain Management Physician), 65, 109
polyetheretherketone, 48
positive attitude, 97, 102
post-acute withdrawal syndrome (PAWS), 75
post-anesthesia care unit (PACU), 55, 108
post-concussion MTBI, 24
post-op. *See also* post-operative.

Index

ACDF adjustment-phase pain, 65
ACDF recovery, 17, 61, 80
ACDF related pain, 65, 66
ACDF surgery pain, 56
  defined, 109
  dysphasia, 55
  first year, 62
  myofascial pain, 77, 78
  pain, 55, 56, 59, 77, 78, 95
post-operative. *See also* post-op.
  care, 11
  complications, 19, 37, 41, 44, 47–50, 54, 58, 62, 95
  fusion success rates, 48–49
  pain, 17
  recovery, 16–17, 20, 54
post-surgery, 57, 65, 68
posture, poor, 97
potassium test, 51
power within yourself, 99
pre-authorization, 89
pre-operative consultation, 50
pre-operative instructions, 50–51
prednisone, 30
pregabalin, 72–73
preparation for ACDF surgery, 101
preparing mentally, 60
prescription pain medication, 18, 24, 25–26, 52, 54, 56–57, 61, 64, 65, 71–76, 94, 95, 104, 105, 110
  abuse of, 64
  addiction to, 64
  avoid taking, 72

primary care physician (PCP), 25, 29–30, 67, 108
privacy, maintaining your, 73
proactive, 72
problems with diagnostic testing, 38
Proceedings of the National Academy of Science, 93
profits for insurance companies, 87, 88
protective gear, 23
protocols, 49, 53
protruding discs, 82
protrusion, 27, 32–33, 36, 42, 66, 105
pseudarthrosis, 16, 19, 48–49, 109
psilocybin, 77
psychoactive chemicals, 77
psychological
  benefits of exercise, 83
  distress, 110
  responses before surgery, 53
  setbacks, 17
  shock, 109
  stress, 52, 58, 101
  support, 68
psychosomatic disorder, 58, 59, 109
psychosomatic perceived limitations, 58
pulmonary aspiration, 53, 109

Q
quality of care, 19
questioning the doctor, 46
questions, 21, 46, 72

final, 50
prior to surgery, 18, 54
right, 12, 18, 21, 46, 90

R
radiating arm pain, 16
radiating pain, 16, 29, 81
radiation, electromagnetic, 110
radiculopathy, 29, 81–82, 109
radiofrequency ablation (RFA), 78–79
radiologist, 20–21, 31, 35, 38–39, 109
  role of, 39
  written report from, 39
range of options, 41
read your policy, 88
records, keeping detailed, 21
recovery
  from ACDF surgery, 16–17, 19–20, 26, 50, 54, 58, 59, 60, 61–62, 80, 82, 83, 94, 98, 101, 102
  likelihood of a full, 62
  phase pain, 94
  speedy, 101
  time, 58, 60
  treatment protocol for, 80
  what to expect during, 19
referred pain, 26, 109
relationships with others, 98
research, informal, 41
residual pain or scarring, 102
respiratory therapist, 20, 106
resulting conditions following ACDF, 20

RFA (radiofrequency ablation), 78–79
rhizotomy, 78
right combination of therapy, 72
risks
  of ACDF surgery, 19–20, 44, 46, 51, 74
  of nerve block injections, 79
  potential, 19
  of taking opioids, 76
rude patients, 57

S
scoliosis (curvature of the spine), 80
second opinion, 42–43, 45–46, 72
security, false sense of, 59
sedentary life after surgery, 99
sedentary lifestyle, 49, 97–98
seizures, 30, 76, 105
sense of community and individual connectedness, 98
sequela, 35
shingles, pain after, 73
shock (defined), 109
showers, cold/hot, 84
sickness as a weakness, 93
side effects
  of chronic pain 68
  of medications, 71, 72, 74
  of opioid medications, 74
  serious, 72
signs and symptoms, 27
sleep deprivation, 61
sleep, 30, 51, 53, 56–57, 61, 73, 83, 101, 103

Index

sleeping pills, 83
specialist, 44, 45–46, 67–68
  advantages and disadvantages of, 67
  referral, 30
spinal canal, 32, 33, 36, 37
spinal column, 16, 110
spinal cord, 29, 32, 35–36, 42, 44, 73, 107
  injury nerve pain, 73
  problems with compressed, 29
spinal fusion chat rooms, 17
spine (defined), 110
spondylodesis/spondylosyndesis, 105
stagnation, 62
stenosis, 27, 33, 37, 72, 82, 110
step-down unit, 54–55
steroid, 30, 67, 79, 90, 105
stigma
  associated with medications, 94
  attached to illness and injury, 93
  of caring for pain-management patients, 67
  of marijuana, 76
stress reaction, acute, 109
stressful event, 109
stretching, 18, 81, 84
stretching exercises for home, 81
success rates, 48–49
sugar, 84, 98
suicide to escape the pain, 66
supplements, 62, 65, 71–72, 74, 84, 108
surgeon, choice of, 41
surgery
  aftermath of, 61, 73
  day after, 57, 60
  fear of, 101
  future, 101
  standard protocol for most, 53
  step-down unit, 55
surgical consultation, 16, 41–43, 45, 47, 49, 51
surgical scars, 18
symptoms
  awareness of, 29
  health-related, 63
  manage your, 71
  signs and, 27

T

T2 sequence, 32, 35
taper-off period, 75
TBI (traumatic brain injury), 110
technology, overuse of, 97
TENS (Transcutaneous Electrical Nerve Stimulation) unit, 85
tension and stress, 27
testing, diagnostic, 38
tetrahydrocannabinol (THC), 76
therapeutic method, 106
therapy, MDT, 80–82
therapy, right combination of, 72
third opinion, 45
tingling sensation, 78, 109
tolerance, building, 74
trauma, 16–17, 23, 26, 104–105, 110
trauma-related injuries, 16
treatment/treatments, 65–66, 82, 84
  alternative, 85, 89

approaches, 41
modalities, types of, 19
non-medication, 77
options, 41, 64, 67, 71, 85
team, 39
tuberculosis, 16
Tylenol, 27, 103

U
unconsciousness (defined), 110
unexpected events, 101
unhealthy food, 50, 98
uninformed patient, 18–19

V
Valium, 52
vertebra/vertebrae, 16, 24, 26, 35–37, 42, 48, 105, 106, 110
vertebral body, 35
vicious cycle, 61, 83
Vicodin (hydrocodone), 25, 74, 110
vitamins, 50, 62

W
war on drugs, 94
water, 55, 101
WBC (White Blood Count), 51
well-being, healthy lifestyle and, 83–84
well-being, psychological, 98–99

X
X-rays, 24, 30–31, 38, 109, 110

Y
yoga, 65, 83–84

Z
Zagata, Dr. Mateusz, 11–12

Acknowledgments

I would like to thank all of those in the medical community directly involved in my care while undergoing ACDF surgery, including the surgeon, anesthesiologist, respiratory therapist, physician's assistant, nurses, staff—and especially my wife, who tended to my care throughout.

I would like to thank Mateusz Zagata, M.D., the family physician who has helped me and my family through sickness and health. Doctor Zagata is a true healer, a man of faith and gifted physician.

I would like to thank my publisher, Maurice Bassett and his wife Ilona, also humanitarians and ambassadors of the world and servants of Divine, who've assisted and encouraged me throughout the writing process.

I would like to thank the editor Chris Nelson for his writing skill and patience while working with a new author unfamiliar with the process. Chris is a humble and compassionate human helping to make the planet a better place.

I would like to thank David Michael Moore, artist and book cover designer for his creative mind and ability to understand his clients' needs and to represent their intent.

As a devout Christian, I would like to thank my Father, God Divine, and his only begotten son Jesus Christ, who sacrificed himself for the faithful, paving a way back to a home, that we, children of the light, may otherwise have been permanently separated from by our sinful nature.

About the Author

Patrick Smith currently resides in Sarasota County Florida, "The Sunshine State," bordering the majestic Myakka State Forest and home to the Florida Panther and Florida Manatee. Patrick considers Florida paradise on Earth (state motto: "In God We Trust").

Patrick moved to Florida after retiring from a career in law enforcement. He is a military veteran and considers himself an ambassador of Christ and servant of God first.

Patrick is married to Jennifer, his wife of thirty years. He is currently a full-time life coach, assisting those in need and specializing in crisis intervention and spiritual guidance.

Having served as a law enforcement officer, federal agent, peer counselor and trained Crisis Intervention Team member, Patrick still remains in close contact with many of those whom he worked with. He assists other law enforcement officers, federal agents, and personal friends in coping with traumatic events, including the loss of loved ones, survivors of suicide and divorce. His work bridges the gap between mental health professionals and those who find themselves with no one to turn to in times of need.

In his spare moments Patrick spends time with his family enjoying the great State of Florida's wildlife, ocean and parks.

You can connect with Patrick at:

www.NeckFusionSurgery.com

Publisher's Catalogue

The Mahatma Gandhi Library

#1 *Towards Non-Violent Politics*

* * *

The Prosperous Series

#1 *The Prosperous Coach: Increase Income and Impact for You and Your Clients* (Steve Chandler and Rich Litvin)

#2 *The Prosperous Hip Hop Producer: My Beat-Making Journey from My Grandma's Patio to a Six-Figure Business* (Curtiss King)

#3 *The Prosperous Hotelier* (David Lund)

* * *

Devon Bandison

Fatherhood Is Leadership: Your Playbook for Success, Self-Leadership, and a Richer Life

Roy G. Biv

Dancing on Antique Toning: A Further Celebration of Numismatic Art

Dancing on Rainbows: A Celebration of Numismatic Art

Sir Fairfax L. Cartwright

The Mystic Rose from the Garden of the King

Steve Chandler

37 Ways to BOOST Your Coaching Practice: PLUS: the 17 Lies That Hold Coaches Back and the Truth That Sets Them Free

50 Ways to Create Great Relationships

Business Coaching (Steve Chandler and Sam Beckford)

Crazy Good: A Book of CHOICES

CREATOR

Death Wish: The Path through Addiction to a Glorious Life

Fearless: Creating the Courage to Change the Things You Can

How to Get Clients (Revised Edition)

The Prosperous Coach: Increase Income and Impact for You and Your Clients (The Prosperous Series #1) (Steve Chandler and Rich Litvin)

RIGHT NOW: Mastering the Beauty of the Present Moment

Shift Your Mind Shift The World (Revised Edition)

Time Warrior: How to defeat procrastination, people-pleasing, self-doubt, over-commitment, broken promises and chaos

Wealth Warrior: The Personal Prosperity Revolution

Kazimierz Dąbrowski

Positive Disintegration

Charles Dickens

A Christmas Carol: A Special Full-Color, Fully-Illustrated Edition

Melissa Ford

Living Service: The Journey of a Prosperous Coach

M. K. Gandhi

Towards Non-Violent Politics (*Mahatma Gandhi Library #1*)

James F. Gesualdi

Excellence Beyond Compliance: Enhancing Animal Welfare Through the Constructive Use of the Animal Welfare Act

Janice Goldman

Let's Talk About Money: The Girlfriends' Guide to Protecting Her ASSets

Sylvia Hall

This Is Real Life: Love Notes to Wake You Up

Christy Harden

Guided by Your Own Stars: Connect with the Inner Voice and Discover Your Dreams

I ♥ Raw: A How-To Guide for Reconnecting to Yourself and the Earth through Plant-Based Living

Curtiss King

The Prosperous Hip Hop Producer: My Beat-Making Journey from My Grandma's Patio to a Six-Figure Business (The Prosperous Series #2)

David Lindsay

A Blade for Sale: The Adventures of Monsieur de Mailly

David Lund

The Prosperous Hotelier (The Prosperous Series #3)

Abraham H. Maslow

The Aims of Education (audio)

The B-language Workshop (audio)

Being Abraham Maslow (DVD)

The Eupsychian Ethic (audio)

The Farther Reaches of Human Nature (audio)

Maslow and Self-Actualization (DVD)

Maslow on Management (audiobook)

Personality and Growth: A Humanistic Psychologist in the Classroom

Psychology and Religious Awareness (audio)

The Psychology of Science: A Reconnaissance

Self-Actualization (audio)

Weekend with Maslow (audio)

Harold E. Robles

Albert Schweitzer: An Adventurer for Humanity

Albert Schweitzer

Reverence for Life: The Words of Albert Schweitzer

Patrick O. Smith

ACDF: The Informed Patient: My journey undergoing neck fusion surgery

William Tillier

Personality Development through Positive Disintegration: The Work of Kazimierz Dąbrowski

Margery Williams

The Velveteen Rabbit: or How Toys Become Real

Join our Mailing List:
www.MauriceBassett.com

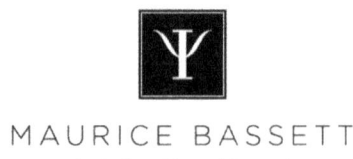

www.ingramcontent.com/pod-product-compliance
Lightning Source LLC
Chambersburg PA
CBHW070051120426
42742CB00048B/2399